THE ULTIMATE

RENAL DIET COOKBOOK

FOR BEGINNERS

I0416143

Complete, Nourishing and Nutritious Recipes with Low-Sodium, Phosphorus and Potassium that helps patients to manage Kidney Disease.

Olivia Endwell

Copyright Statement:

Disclaimer:

The information provided in this book is for educational and informational purposes only. It is not intended as a substitute for professional medical advice, diagnosis, or treatment. Always seek the advice of your physician or other qualified health provider with any questions you may have regarding a medical condition. Never disregard professional medical advice or delay in seeking it because of something you have read in this book.

The author and publisher disclaim any liability arising directly or indirectly from the use of this book. The information provided is based on the author's best knowledge at the time of writing and is subject to change. The author and publisher do not guarantee the accuracy, completeness, or timeliness of the information presented in this book.

Individual results may vary, and the success of any dietary or lifestyle change depends on various factors, including but not limited to individual commitment and adherence. Before making significant changes to your diet or lifestyle, consult with a qualified healthcare professional.

The views and opinions expressed in this book are those of the author and do not necessarily reflect the official policy or position of any other agency, organization, employer, or company.

TABLE OF CONTENTS

INTRODUCTION

Welcome to "The Ultimate Renal Diet Cookbook for Beginners" – your essential guide to embracing a healthier lifestyle for optimal kidney function. In this introduction, we'll delve into the fundamental aspects that lay the foundation for our culinary journey through renal wellness.

First and foremost, let's unravel the intricacies of renal health. Your kidneys, those unsung heroes in your body, play a crucial role in filtering waste and maintaining a delicate balance of fluids and electrolytes. Understanding the basics of how these vital organs function is the key to safeguarding your overall well-being.

The food we consume directly impacts the health of our kidneys. A renal-friendly diet isn't just a dietary choice; it's a powerful tool in managing kidney health. By making informed and intentional choices about what we eat, we can support our kidneys, potentially mitigating the risk of complications and fostering a healthier, more vibrant life.

You might be wondering, "Is a renal diet relevant to me?" Whether you're someone managing a kidney condition, concerned about preventing kidney issues, or simply seeking to adopt a health-conscious approach to your diet, this cookbook is designed for you. Discover how small changes in your eating habits can make a significant impact on your renal well-being.

Now, let's talk about what makes this cookbook the ultimate companion on your renal health journey. More than just a collection of recipes, this guide is a comprehensive resource filled with practical tips, nutritional insights, and delicious, kidney-friendly meals. It's crafted with beginners in mind, ensuring that the path to a renal-friendly lifestyle is not only beneficial but also enjoyable.

As you embark on this culinary adventure, remember that every meal is an opportunity to nurture your kidneys and enhance your overall health. So, let's dive in, explore the world of renal-friendly cuisine, and savor the flavors of a life well-nourished.

RENAL DIET FUNDAMENTALS

Basics of Renal Nutrition

Understanding the basics of renal nutrition is fundamental to managing kidney health effectively. The kidneys play a vital role in filtering waste products and excess fluids from the blood, helping maintain a delicate balance of electrolytes. A renal diet, tailored to support these functions, is essential for individuals with kidney conditions or those looking to prevent kidney issues.

The cornerstone of renal nutrition is controlling the intake of certain nutrients. Sodium, potassium, phosphorus, and protein are key players in this dietary approach. Monitoring these elements helps alleviate the strain on the kidneys, promoting overall well-being.

Sodium: The Stealthy Culprit

Sodium, commonly found in table salt and processed foods, can wreak havoc on kidney health when consumed in excess. A renal diet restricts sodium intake to manage blood pressure and reduce fluid retention. Embracing fresh, whole foods and avoiding high-sodium processed options are crucial steps in maintaining a kidney-friendly sodium balance.

Potassium: Balancing Act

While potassium is essential for nerve and muscle function, excessive levels can be harmful to individuals with compromised kidney function. A renal diet carefully regulates potassium intake, emphasizing portion control and selecting low-potassium alternatives. Balancing potassium-rich fruits and vegetables with moderation is the key to supporting kidney health.

Phosphorus: The Hidden Challenge

Phosphorus, abundant in many foods, can be challenging to manage for those with kidney issues. Elevated phosphorus levels contribute to bone and cardiovascular complications. Renal nutrition involves choosing low-phosphorus foods, including dairy alternatives, lean meats, and vegetables, while avoiding high-phosphorus items like processed foods and certain grains.

Protein: Moderation is Key

Protein is essential for body repair and maintenance, but excessive protein intake can strain the kidneys. A renal diet focuses on moderating protein consumption while ensuring adequate nutrition. High-quality protein sources, such as lean meats, fish, eggs, and plant-based options, are emphasized to strike the right balance between protein needs and kidney health.

Nutrients to Monitor

In the realm of renal diet fundamentals, vigilant monitoring of specific nutrients is paramount. The interplay between sodium, potassium, phosphorus, and protein requires a nuanced approach to ensure optimal kidney function.

Balancing Act: Sodium and Potassium

The delicate balance between sodium and potassium is crucial for kidney health. Excessive sodium intake can lead to elevated blood pressure and fluid retention, while inadequate potassium levels may impact muscle and nerve function. A renal diet meticulously regulates the intake of these minerals, promoting a harmonious equilibrium that supports overall kidney function.

Navigating Phosphorus: A Strategic Approach

Phosphorus management is a strategic aspect of renal nutrition. While essential for bone health, elevated phosphorus levels can contribute to cardiovascular complications in individuals with kidney issues. Monitoring and limiting phosphorus-rich foods are key components of a renal diet, fostering a proactive approach to safeguarding kidney health.

Protein Moderation: A Comprehensive View

Protein moderation is not just about quantity but also quality. A renal diet encourages the consumption of high-quality protein sources while moderating overall protein intake. This comprehensive approach ensures that the body receives essential amino acids without overburdening the kidneys, promoting a balanced and sustainable dietary pattern.

Importance of Fluid Balance

Fluid balance is a critical aspect of renal health often overlooked in mainstream nutrition discussions. The kidneys play a central role in regulating fluid levels in the body, and individuals with kidney issues need to be particularly mindful of their fluid intake.

The Kidneys' Fluid Regulation Dance

The kidneys' primary function involves filtering waste and excess fluids from the blood. Maintaining an intricate dance of fluid balance is vital for overall health. In renal conditions, the kidneys' ability to regulate fluid balance may be compromised, leading to fluid retention or dehydration. A renal diet takes into account individual fluid needs, striking a delicate balance to support optimal kidney function.

Fluid Intake Guidelines: Tailoring to Individual Needs

Guidelines for fluid intake in a renal diet are not one-size-fits-all. Factors such as age, weight, activity level, and the stage of kidney disease play a role in determining individual fluid needs. A personalized approach ensures that individuals with kidney issues receive the right amount of fluids to maintain hydration without overburdening the kidneys.

Detecting Fluid Imbalances: Signs and Symptoms

Understanding the signs and symptoms of fluid imbalances is crucial for individuals managing kidney conditions. Swelling (edema), changes in urine output, and blood pressure fluctuations can indicate fluid retention or dehydration. A renal diet, in conjunction with regular monitoring and medical guidance, helps individuals detect and address fluid imbalances promptly.

Reading Food Labels for Renal Health

Navigating the aisles of the grocery store becomes a skill in itself when following a renal diet. Reading food labels becomes a powerful tool for making informed choices and maintaining optimal kidney health.

Decoding Sodium Content: The Fine Print

Sodium content is often hidden in processed foods under various names. Learning to decode food labels for sodium content is crucial in a renal diet. Ingredients like monosodium glutamate (MSG), baking soda, and sodium benzoate may contribute to elevated sodium intake. Renal-conscious consumers become adept at identifying and choosing low-sodium alternatives, promoting kidney-friendly eating habits.

Unraveling Phosphorus Mysteries: Ingredient Awareness

Phosphorus additives lurk in unexpected places, such as preservatives and flavor enhancers. Reading food labels with an eye for phosphorus-containing additives helps individuals with kidney issues avoid hidden sources of this mineral. A renal diet encourages a discerning approach, empowering individuals to make choices that align with their nutritional needs and support kidney health.

Protein Portioning: Quantifying Quality

Protein content and source are pivotal considerations when reading food labels on a renal diet. Understanding the protein needs for individual health and selecting foods with high-quality protein sources become second nature. A renal-conscious consumer learns to identify and prioritize foods that contribute to overall well-being without compromising kidney health.

GETTING STARTED WITH THE RENAL DIET

Embarking on a renal diet is a transformative journey that involves thoughtful consideration and proactive planning. In this comprehensive guide, we will explore the essential steps to initiate your renal diet successfully.

Assessing Your Dietary Needs

The first and crucial step in adopting a renal diet is a thorough assessment of your dietary needs. This involves understanding your overall health, kidney function, and any specific dietary restrictions or recommendations provided by your healthcare team.

Understanding Your Health Profile

To tailor a renal diet to your needs, it's essential to have a comprehensive understanding of your health profile. This includes factors such as your current kidney function, any pre-existing medical conditions, medications you may be taking, and your overall nutritional status. Gathering this information provides a solid foundation for crafting a personalized and effective renal diet plan.

Tracking Kidney Function: Laboratory Tests

Laboratory tests, such as serum creatinine, blood urea nitrogen (BUN), and glomerular filtration rate (GFR), offer valuable insights into your kidney function. Regular monitoring of these markers allows healthcare professionals to assess the progression of kidney disease and guide adjustments to your renal diet. Understanding your lab results empowers you to actively participate in managing your kidney health.

Consulting with Healthcare Professionals

A collaborative approach with healthcare professionals is indispensable when adopting a renal diet. These professionals, including nephrologists, dietitians, and other specialists, play a pivotal role in guiding you through the intricacies of renal nutrition.

Building a Supportive Healthcare Team

Establishing a healthcare team dedicated to renal health is crucial. Nephrologists specialize in kidney care and can provide insights into the specific needs of your kidneys. Dietitians with expertise in renal nutrition offer personalized guidance, ensuring your dietary choices align with your health goals. Collaborating with these professionals creates a supportive framework for your renal diet journey.

Regular Check-ins and Adjustments

The journey of adopting a renal diet is dynamic, with your health status evolving over time. Regular check-ins with your healthcare team facilitate ongoing assessment and adjustments to your renal diet plan. This proactive approach ensures that your dietary choices remain aligned with your changing health needs, promoting optimal kidney function and overall well-being.

Kitchen Essentials for Renal Cooking

Equipping your kitchen with the right tools and ingredients is a practical and empowering step in embracing a renal diet. Renal-friendly cooking involves thoughtful preparation and an understanding of ingredients that support kidney health.

Stocking a Kidney-Friendly Pantry

Building a kidney-friendly pantry involves selecting ingredients that align with the principles of a renal diet. Opting for low-sodium broths, whole grains, fresh fruits and vegetables, and lean protein sources ensures that your pantry is stocked with nutritious and kidney-friendly options. This not only simplifies meal preparation but also promotes consistent adherence to your renal diet.

Investing in Quality Cookware

Investing in quality cookware is an often-overlooked aspect of renal-friendly cooking. Non-stick pans, for example, reduce the need for excessive fats or oils, promoting heart-healthy cooking practices. Choosing utensils that are easy to clean and maintain ensures that cooking remains an enjoyable and hassle-free experience.

Meal Prep Tools for Efficiency

Efficient meal preparation is a key component of sustaining a renal diet. Investing in tools such as a sharp knife, cutting boards, and storage containers streamlines the cooking process, making it easier to incorporate renal-friendly meals into your daily routine. These tools not only save time but also contribute to the overall success of your renal diet journey.

Planning Renal-Friendly Meals

Planning is at the heart of a successful renal diet. From understanding portion sizes to creating balanced meals, thoughtful planning sets the stage for a sustainable and enjoyable dietary approach.

Portion Control: Finding the Right Balance

Portion control is a fundamental aspect of a renal diet, especially concerning protein, sodium, and phosphorus. Understanding appropriate portion sizes helps manage nutrient intake without overburdening the kidneys. This skill becomes second nature with practice, ensuring that your meals are not only kidney-friendly but also delicious and satisfying.

Balanced Plate Approach

Adopting a balanced plate approach involves incorporating a variety of nutrient-dense foods into your meals. This includes a mix of fruits, vegetables, whole grains, and lean proteins. Striking a balance among different food groups ensures that your body receives the necessary nutrients while maintaining the principles of a renal diet.

Creating Weekly Meal Plans

Weekly meal planning simplifies the process of adhering to a renal diet. Planning ahead allows you to select recipes, create shopping lists, and ensure a diverse and well-rounded menu. This proactive approach minimizes stress and supports consistent adherence to your renal diet, fostering a sustainable and positive dietary experience.

BEVERAGES FOR KIDNEY HEALTH

The role of beverages in kidney health is often underestimated, yet their impact on the kidneys is profound. In this exploration of "Beverages for Kidney Health," we delve into the importance of hydration, the array of kidney-friendly drink choices, and the art of crafting refreshing beverages at home – all essential elements for supporting optimal kidney function.

Importance of Hydration

Hydration is the cornerstone of kidney health, and its significance extends far beyond quenching thirst. The kidneys, responsible for filtering waste and excess fluids from the blood, rely on adequate hydration to perform their vital functions effectively.

The Kidneys' Hydration Dance

Imagine your kidneys as meticulous choreographers orchestrating a hydration dance within your body. Their primary mission is to maintain a delicate balance of fluids and electrolytes, ensuring that waste is efficiently eliminated while essential nutrients are retained. Optimal hydration supports this intricate dance, promoting the kidneys' ability to filter blood and regulate various bodily functions.

Fluids as Kidney Allies

Ample fluid intake acts as a steadfast ally for your kidneys. Water, the elixir of life, is the primary choice for hydration, but other kidney-friendly fluids play crucial roles as well. Herbal teas, clear broths, and certain fruit juices contribute to overall fluid intake without imposing undue stress on the kidneys. Understanding the diverse options available empowers individuals to tailor their beverage choices to both preference and kidney health.

Hydration and Kidney Stones Prevention

Adequate hydration is a formidable weapon in the prevention of kidney stones, a painful condition caused by the crystallization of minerals in the urine. Diluted urine, achieved through proper hydration, helps inhibit the formation of these crystals. By consistently meeting your body's fluid needs, you create an environment that discourages the development of kidney stones, safeguarding your renal health.

Kidney-Friendly Drink Choices

Not all beverages are created equal when it comes to kidney health. Making informed choices about what you drink can significantly impact your overall well-being. Let's explore kidney-friendly drink choices that not only hydrate but also support optimal kidney function.

Water: Nature's Perfect Elixir

Water stands as the epitome of kidney-friendly hydration. It is pure, calorie-free, and essential for the kidneys' filtration process. Regular water consumption helps prevent dehydration, reduces the risk of kidney stones, and supports overall kidney function. Making water your primary beverage choice is a simple yet powerful step towards maintaining renal health.

Herbal Teas: Infusions of Wellness

Herbal teas, devoid of caffeine, provide a flavorful alternative to water while contributing to your daily fluid intake. Certain herbal teas, such as nettle tea, may even offer potential benefits for kidney health. Their hydrating properties, coupled with antioxidant-rich profiles, make herbal teas a delightful and kidney-friendly addition to your beverage repertoire.

Clear Broths: Nourishing Hydration

Clear broths, whether vegetable or bone-based, offer a dual advantage of hydration and nourishment. Low in phosphorus and sodium, clear broths provide a comforting and kidney-friendly option. Enjoying a warm cup of clear broth not only contributes to your fluid intake but also adds a savory touch to your dietary routine, supporting both hydration and overall well-being.

Fruit Juices in Moderation: A Refreshing Indulgence

While water remains the optimal choice, moderate consumption of certain fruit juices can be incorporated into a renal-friendly diet. Choose juices that are lower in potassium and phosphorus, and be mindful of portion sizes to avoid excessive sugar intake. Diluting juices with water or opting for homemade varieties allows you to savor the flavors while maintaining a kidney-conscious approach.

Crafting Refreshing Beverages at Home

The allure of crafting refreshing beverages at home lies not only in the joy of creativity but also in the ability to tailor drinks to meet specific dietary needs. Let's explore the art of concocting kidney-friendly beverages within the comfort of your own kitchen.

Homemade Infusions: Flavorful and Kidney-Friendly

Infusing water with fresh fruits, herbs, or vegetables adds a burst of flavor to your hydration routine. Citrus slices, cucumber, mint, or berries not only enhance the taste but also provide additional nutrients without compromising kidney health. Experimenting with different combinations allows you to discover personalized infusions that make hydration a delightful experience.

DIY Herbal Tea Blends: Customized Wellness in a Cup

Crafting your own herbal tea blends opens the door to a world of flavors and potential health benefits. Combine herbs like chamomile, peppermint, and dandelion for a soothing and kidney-friendly brew. Experimenting with ratios allows you to tailor your tea to suit your taste preferences while supporting your kidneys with every sip.

Smoothies for Nutrient Boosts

Smoothies offer a versatile canvas for creating kidney-friendly, nutrient-packed beverages. Blend fruits like berries, which are lower in potassium, with non-dairy milk or water for a delicious and hydrating treat. Adding a handful of spinach or kale introduces an extra dose of vitamins without compromising your renal diet. The possibilities are endless, making smoothies a customizable and kidney-conscious option.

Iced Teas and Coffees: Cool Indulgences

For those who relish the cool embrace of iced beverages, crafting kidney-friendly iced teas and coffees at home provides a healthier alternative to commercially available options. Use low-phosphorus teas, avoid excessive sugar, and choose non-dairy milk to create refreshing iced beverages that align with your renal health goals.

Snack Recipes

1. Cucumber and Hummus Bites

Prep Time: 10 minutes

Cooking Time: 0 minutes

Serving Size: 4

Ingredients:

- 1 cucumber, sliced into rounds

- 1/2 cup low-sodium hummus

- Fresh dill for garnish

Instructions:

1. Wash and slice the cucumber into rounds.

2. Spoon a small amount of hummus onto each cucumber slice.

3. Garnish with fresh dill.

4. Serve immediately and enjoy this refreshing, kidney-friendly snack.

Nutritional Information (per serving):

- Calories: 70

- Protein: 3g

- Sodium: 110mg

- Potassium: 150mg

- Phosphorus: 60mg

2. Baked Sweet Potato Chips

Prep Time: 15 minutes
Cooking Time: 25 minutes
Serving Size: 2

Ingredients:

- 1 large sweet potato, thinly sliced

- 1 tablespoon olive oil

- 1/2 teaspoon garlic powder

- 1/2 teaspoon paprika

- Salt to taste

Instructions:

1. Preheat the oven to 375°F (190°C).

2. In a bowl, toss sweet potato slices with olive oil, garlic powder, paprika, and salt.

3. Arrange slices on a baking sheet in a single layer.

4. Bake for 20-25 minutes until crisp, flipping halfway through.

5. Let cool before serving.

Nutritional Information (per serving):

- Calories: 120

- Protein: 2g

- Sodium: 90mg

- Potassium: 200mg

- Phosphorus: 40mg

3. Berry Yogurt Parfait

Prep Time: 10 minutes
Cooking Time: 0 minutes
Serving Size: 1

Ingredients:

- 1/2 cup low-fat vanilla yogurt

- 1/4 cup fresh blueberries

- 1/4 cup fresh strawberries, sliced

- 2 tablespoons granola (low-phosphorus)

Instructions:

1. In a glass or bowl, layer half of the yogurt.

2. Add half of the blueberries and strawberries.

3. Sprinkle a tablespoon of granola.

4. Repeat the layers.

5. Serve immediately and savor this delightful kidney-friendly treat.

Nutritional Information (per serving):

- Calories: 220

- Protein: 8g

- Sodium: 80mg

- Potassium: 180mg

- Phosphorus: 80mg

4. Avocado and Tomato Salsa with Whole Grain Pita

Prep Time: 15 minutes
Cooking Time: 0 minutes
Serving Size: 2

Ingredients:

- 1 ripe avocado, diced

- 1 cup cherry tomatoes, halved

- 1/4 cup red onion, finely chopped

- 1 tablespoon fresh cilantro, chopped

- Juice of 1 lime

- 2 whole grain pitas, cut into wedges

Instructions:

1. In a bowl, combine diced avocado, cherry tomatoes, red onion, cilantro, and lime juice.

2. Mix well and let it sit for 5 minutes to allow flavors to meld.

3. Toast whole grain pita wedges.

4. Serve the avocado and tomato salsa with the pita wedges.

Nutritional Information (per serving):

- Calories: 240

- Protein: 5g

- Sodium: 200mg

- Potassium: 400mg

- Phosphorus: 80mg

5. Greek Yogurt and Cucumber Dip with Veggie Sticks

Prep Time: 15 minutes
Cooking Time: 0 minutes
Serving Size: 4

Ingredients:

- 1 cup Greek yogurt

- 1/2 cucumber, finely diced

- 1 tablespoon fresh dill, chopped

- 1 clove garlic, minced

- Assorted vegetable sticks (carrots, bell peppers, celery)

Instructions:

1. In a bowl, combine Greek yogurt, diced cucumber, dill, and minced garlic.

2. Mix well and refrigerate for at least 10 minutes.

3. Prepare assorted vegetable sticks.

4. Serve the Greek yogurt and cucumber dip with the vegetable sticks.

Nutritional Information (per serving):

- Calories: 80

- Protein: 6g

- Sodium: 40mg

- Potassium: 180mg

- Phosphorus: 60mg

6. Tuna Salad Lettuce Wraps

Prep Time: 15 minutes
Cooking Time: 0 minutes
Serving Size: 2

Ingredients:

- 1 can (5 ounces) low-sodium tuna, drained

- 2 tablespoons mayonnaise (low-phosphorus)

- 1 celery stalk, finely chopped

- 1 tablespoon red onion, finely chopped

- 1 teaspoon Dijon mustard

- 4 large lettuce leaves

Instructions:

1. In a bowl, mix tuna, mayonnaise, chopped celery, red onion, and Dijon mustard.

2. Spoon the tuna salad onto lettuce leaves.

3. Roll the lettuce leaves to form wraps.

4. Secure with toothpicks and serve.

Nutritional Information (per serving):

- Calories: 180

- Protein: 15g

- Sodium: 220mg

- Potassium: 200mg

- Phosphorus: 120mg

7. Roasted Chickpeas

Prep Time: 10 minutes

Cooking Time: 30 minutes

Serving Size: 4

Ingredients:

- 1 can (15 ounces) chickpeas, drained and rinsed

- 1 tablespoon olive oil

- 1/2 teaspoon cumin

- 1/2 teaspoon paprika

- 1/2 teaspoon garlic powder

- Salt to taste

Instructions:

1. Preheat the oven to 400°F (200°C).

2. Pat chickpeas dry with a paper towel.

3. In a bowl, toss chickpeas with olive oil, cumin, paprika, garlic powder, and salt.

4. Spread chickpeas on a baking sheet and roast for 30 minutes, stirring halfway through.

5. Let cool before serving.

Nutritional Information (per serving):

- Calories: 140

- Protein: 6g

- Sodium: 230mg

- Potassium: 100mg

- Phosphorus: 60mg

8. Cottage Cheese and Pineapple Skewers

Prep Time: 10 minutes

Cooking Time: 0 minutes

Serving Size: 2

Ingredients:

- 1 cup low-fat cottage cheese

- 1 cup fresh pineapple, cubed

- Wooden skewers

Instructions:

1. Alternate threading cubes of cottage cheese and pineapple onto wooden skewers.

2. Serve immediately for a delightful and protein-rich snack.

Nutritional Information (per serving):

- Calories: 160

- Protein: 15g

- Sodium: 320mg

- Potassium: 180mg

- Phosphorus: 120mg

9. Apple and Almond Butter Slices

Prep Time: 10 minutes
Cooking Time: 0 minutes
Serving Size: 2

Ingredients:

- 1 apple, sliced

- 4 tablespoons almond butter (unsalted)

Instructions:

1. Slice the apple into thin rounds.

2. Spread almond butter on each apple slice.

3. Arrange the slices on a plate and enjoy this simple yet satisfying kidney-friendly snack.

Nutritional Information (per serving):

- Calories: 220

- Protein: 5g

- Sodium: 5mg

- Potassium: 180mg

- Phosphorus: 80mg

10. Quinoa Salad Cups

Prep Time: 20 minutes

Cooking Time: 15 minutes

Serving Size: 4

Ingredients:

- 1 cup cooked quinoa
- 1/2 cup cucumber, diced
- 1/2 cup cherry tomatoes, halved
- 1/4 cup feta cheese (low-phosphorus), crumbled
- 2 tablespoons fresh basil, chopped
- 2 tablespoons balsamic vinaigrette

Instructions:

1. In a bowl, combine cooked quinoa, diced cucumber, cherry tomatoes, feta cheese, and fresh basil.

2. Drizzle with balsamic vinaigrette and toss to combine.

3. Spoon the quinoa salad into small cups for a convenient and nutritious snack.

Nutritional Information (per serving):

- Calories: 180
- Protein: 6g

- Sodium: 180mg

- Potassium: 220mg

- Phosphorus: 90mg

BREAKFAST RECIPES

1. Quinoa Breakfast Bowl

Prep Time: 10 minutes

Cooking Time: 15 minutes

Serving Size: 2

Ingredients:

- 1 cup cooked quinoa

- 1/2 cup fresh berries (blueberries, strawberries)

- 2 tablespoons chopped almonds

- 1 tablespoon honey

- 1/2 teaspoon cinnamon

Instructions:

1. In a bowl, combine cooked quinoa, fresh berries, and chopped almonds.

2. Drizzle with honey and sprinkle cinnamon.

3. Mix well and serve for a protein-packed and delicious breakfast.

Nutritional Information (per serving):

- Calories: 300

- Protein: 8g

- Sodium: 10mg

- Potassium: 220mg

- Phosphorus: 150mg

2. Veggie Omelette with Spinach and Feta

Prep Time: 10 minutes

Cooking Time: 10 minutes

Serving Size: 1

Ingredients:

- 2 large eggs

- 1/4 cup spinach, chopped

- 2 tablespoons feta cheese (low-phosphorus), crumbled

- 1/4 cup bell peppers, diced

- Salt and pepper to taste

Instructions:

1. Whisk eggs in a bowl and season with salt and pepper.

2. In a non-stick pan, sauté spinach and bell peppers until tender.

3. Pour whisked eggs over the veggies and cook until set.

4. Sprinkle feta cheese over one half, fold, and serve.

Nutritional Information (per serving):

- Calories: 220

- Protein: 17g

- Sodium: 320mg

- Potassium: 200mg

- Phosphorus: 180mg

3. Overnight Chia Seed Pudding

Prep Time: 5 minutes (plus overnight refrigeration)

Cooking Time: 0 minutes

Serving Size: 1

Ingredients:

- 2 tablespoons chia seeds

- 1/2 cup almond milk (unsweetened)

- 1/2 teaspoon vanilla extract

- 1 tablespoon sliced almonds

- Fresh berries for topping

Instructions:

1. In a jar, mix chia seeds, almond milk, and vanilla extract.

2. Refrigerate overnight.

3. Before serving, top with sliced almonds and fresh berries.

Nutritional Information (per serving):

- Calories: 180

- Protein: 5g

- Sodium: 80mg

- Potassium: 120mg

- Phosphorus: 80mg

4. Banana Walnut Pancakes

Prep Time: 15 minutes

Cooking Time: 10 minutes

Serving Size: 2

Ingredients:

- 1 ripe banana, mashed

- 2 large eggs

- 1/2 cup whole wheat flour

- 1/4 cup chopped walnuts

- 1/2 teaspoon baking powder

- 1/2 teaspoon cinnamon

- Maple syrup for drizzling

Instructions:

1. In a bowl, mash the banana and whisk in eggs.

2. Add whole wheat flour, chopped walnuts, baking powder, and cinnamon. Mix until smooth.

3. Heat a non-stick pan and ladle the batter to make pancakes.

4. Cook until bubbles form, flip, and cook the other side.

5. Drizzle with maple syrup before serving.

Nutritional Information (per serving):

- Calories: 320

- Protein: 12g

- Sodium: 80mg

- Potassium: 340mg

- Phosphorus: 160mg

5. Greek Yogurt Parfait with Granola

Prep Time: 10 minutes

Cooking Time: 0 minutes

Serving Size: 1

Ingredients:

- 1/2 cup low-fat Greek yogurt

- 1/4 cup granola (low-phosphorus)

- 1/4 cup fresh berries (raspberries, blackberries)

Instructions:

1. In a glass, layer Greek yogurt, granola, and fresh berries.

2. Repeat the layers.

3. Serve immediately for a protein-rich and satisfying breakfast.

Nutritional Information (per serving):

- Calories: 250

- Protein: 15g

- Sodium: 50mg

- Potassium: 180mg

- Phosphorus: 120mg

6. Spinach and Mushroom Frittata

Prep Time: 15 minutes
Cooking Time: 20 minutes
Serving Size: 4

Ingredients:

- 6 large eggs

- 1 cup spinach, chopped

- 1/2 cup mushrooms, sliced

- 1/4 cup feta cheese (low-phosphorus), crumbled

- 1/4 cup onion, finely chopped

- Salt and pepper to taste

Instructions:

1. Preheat the oven to 350°F (175°C).

2. In a bowl, whisk eggs and season with salt and pepper.

3. Sauté spinach, mushrooms, and onion in an oven-proof pan.

4. Pour whisked eggs over the vegetables, sprinkle feta cheese, and bake until set.

Nutritional Information (per serving):

- Calories: 220

- Protein: 16g

- Sodium: 290mg

- Potassium: 280mg

- Phosphorus: 220mg

7. Blueberry Almond Smoothie Bowl

Prep Time: 10 minutes
Cooking Time: 0 minutes
Serving Size: 1

Ingredients:

- 1/2 cup frozen blueberries

- 1/2 banana, frozen

- 1/2 cup almond milk (unsweetened)

- 2 tablespoons almond butter (unsalted)

- 1 tablespoon chia seeds

Instructions:

1. Blend frozen blueberries, frozen banana, almond milk, and almond butter until smooth.

2. Pour into a bowl and top with chia seeds.

3. Enjoy this nutrient-packed and refreshing smoothie bowl.

Nutritional Information (per serving):

- Calories: 320

- Protein: 9g

- Sodium: 80mg

- Potassium: 400mg

- Phosphorus: 160mg

8. Egg and Vegetable Breakfast Wrap

Prep Time: 15 minutes
Cooking Time: 10 minutes
Serving Size: 1

Ingredients:

- 1 whole grain wrap

- 2 large eggs, scrambled

- 1/4 cup bell peppers, diced

- 1/4 cup tomatoes, diced

- 2 tablespoons low-fat cheese, shredded

- Salsa for topping

Instructions:

1. In a pan, scramble eggs and sauté bell peppers and tomatoes.

2. Place the egg mixture onto a whole grain wrap.

3. Sprinkle shredded cheese and top with salsa.

4. Roll up the wrap and serve.

Nutritional Information (per serving):

- Calories: 350

- Protein: 20g

- Sodium: 480mg

- Potassium: 240mg

- Phosphorus: 220mg

9. Apple Cinnamon Oatmeal

Prep Time: 5 minutes

Cooking Time: 10 minutes

Serving Size: 1

Ingredients:

- 1/2 cup old-fashioned oats

- 1 cup water

- 1/2 apple, diced

- 1/2 teaspoon cinnamon

- 1 tablespoon honey

Instructions:

1. In a pot, combine oats and water. Cook over medium heat.

2. Add diced apples and cinnamon, stirring occasionally.

3. Once cooked, drizzle with honey before serving.

Nutritional Information (per serving):

- Calories: 280

- Protein: 5g

- Sodium: 10mg

- Potassium: 160mg

- Phosphorus: 90mg

10. Whole Grain Bagel with Smoked Salmon

Prep Time: 10 minutes

Cooking Time: 0 minutes

Serving Size: 1

Ingredients:

- 1 whole grain bagel

- 2 tablespoons cream cheese

- 2 ounces smoked salmon

- Capers and red onion slices for topping

Instructions:

1. Toast the whole grain bagel to your liking.

2. Spread cream cheese on each half.

3. Layer with smoked salmon, capers, and red onion slices.

4. Enjoy this savory and protein-rich breakfast.

Nutritional Information (per serving):

- Calories: 380

- Protein: 18g

- Sodium: 520mg

- Potassium: 220mg

- Phosphorus: 160mg

11. Sweet Potato Hash with Turkey Sausage

Prep Time: 15 minutes

Cooking Time: 20 minutes

Serving Size: 2

Ingredients:

- 1 sweet potato, diced

- 1/2 pound lean turkey sausage, crumbled

- 1/2 bell pepper, diced

- 1/4 cup onion, finely chopped

- 1 tablespoon olive oil

- Salt and pepper to taste

Instructions:

1. In a pan, sauté sweet potatoes in olive oil until tender.

2. Add turkey sausage, bell pepper, and onion. Cook until sausage is browned.

3. Season with salt and pepper before serving.

Nutritional Information (per serving):

- Calories: 320

- Protein: 15g

- Sodium: 380mg

- Potassium: 400mg

- Phosphorus: 180mg

12. Chocolate Banana Protein Smoothie

Prep Time: 5 minutes

Cooking Time: 0 minutes

Serving Size: 1

Ingredients:

- 1 ripe banana

- 1 cup unsweetened almond milk

- 1 scoop chocolate protein powder

- 1 tablespoon almond butter (unsalted)

- Ice cubes (optional)

Instructions:

1. In a blender, combine ripe banana, almond milk, chocolate protein powder, and almond butter.

2. Blend until smooth and creamy.

3. Add ice cubes if desired and blend again.

4. Pour into a glass and savor this protein-packed chocolate delight.

Nutritional Information (per serving):

- Calories: 300

- Protein: 20g

- Sodium: 280mg

- Potassium: 470mg

- Phosphorus: 220mg

13. Almond Flour Pancakes

Prep Time: 10 minutes
Cooking Time: 10 minutes
Serving Size: 2

Ingredients:

- 1 cup almond flour

- 2 large eggs

- 1/2 cup almond milk (unsweetened)

- 1/2 teaspoon baking powder

- 1/2 teaspoon vanilla extract

- Fresh berries for topping

Instructions:

1. In a bowl, mix almond flour, eggs, almond milk, baking powder, and vanilla extract until smooth.

2. Heat a non-stick pan and ladle the batter to make pancakes.

3. Cook until bubbles form, flip, and cook the other side.

4. Top with fresh berries before serving.

Nutritional Information (per serving):

- Calories: 380

- Protein: 15g

- Sodium: 150mg

- Potassium: 220mg

- Phosphorus: 160mg

14. Breakfast Burrito with Black Beans and Avocado

Prep Time: 15 minutes
Cooking Time: 10 minutes
Serving Size: 1

Ingredients:

- 1 whole grain tortilla

- 2 large eggs, scrambled

- 1/4 cup black beans, cooked

- 1/4 avocado, sliced

- Salsa for topping

Instructions:

1. In a pan, scramble eggs until cooked.

2. Warm the whole grain tortilla.

3. Layer the tortilla with scrambled eggs, black beans, avocado slices, and salsa.

4. Roll up the burrito and serve.

Nutritional Information (per serving):

- Calories: 350

- Protein: 18g

- Sodium: 450mg

- Potassium: 420mg

- Phosphorus: 240mg

15. Raspberry Coconut Chia Pudding

Prep Time: 5 minutes (plus overnight refrigeration)
Cooking Time: 0 minutes
Serving Size: 1

Ingredients:

- 3 tablespoons chia seeds

- 1/2 cup coconut milk (unsweetened)

- 1/2 cup fresh raspberries

- 1 tablespoon shredded coconut (unsweetened)

Instructions:

1. In a jar, combine chia seeds and coconut milk.

2. Refrigerate overnight.

3. Before serving, top with fresh raspberries and shredded coconut.

Nutritional Information (per serving):

- Calories: 280

- Protein: 7g

- Sodium: 10mg

- Potassium: 160mg

- Phosphorus: 120mg

16. Whole Grain Waffles with Peach Compote

Prep Time: 15 minutes

Cooking Time: 10 minutes

Serving Size: 2

Ingredients:

- 1 cup whole grain waffle mix

- 1 cup water

- 2 peaches, peeled and diced

- 1 tablespoon honey

- 1/2 teaspoon cinnamon

Instructions:

1. Prepare whole grain waffle mix with water according to package instructions.

2. In a pan, simmer diced peaches with honey and cinnamon until softened.

3. Serve waffles with warm peach compote.

Nutritional Information (per serving):

- Calories: 320

- Protein: 8g

- Sodium: 380mg

- Potassium: 300mg

- Phosphorus: 180mg

17. Mediterranean Breakfast Bowl

Prep Time: 10 minutes
Cooking Time: 0 minutes
Serving Size: 1

Ingredients:

- 1/2 cup cooked quinoa

- 1/4 cup cherry tomatoes, halved

- 2 tablespoons feta cheese (low-phosphorus), crumbled

- 1 tablespoon Kalamata olives, sliced

- 1/4 cup cucumber, diced

- 1 tablespoon olive oil

- Fresh parsley for garnish

Instructions:

1. In a bowl, combine cooked quinoa, cherry tomatoes, feta cheese, Kalamata olives, and cucumber.

2. Drizzle with olive oil and garnish with fresh parsley.

3. Enjoy this Mediterranean-inspired breakfast bowl.

Nutritional Information (per serving):

- Calories: 280

- Protein: 8g

- Sodium: 240mg

- Potassium: 230mg

- Phosphorus: 160mg

18. Turkey and Vegetable Breakfast Skillet

Prep Time: 15 minutes

Cooking Time: 15 minutes

Serving Size: 2

Ingredients:

- 1/2 pound lean ground turkey

- 1/2 cup bell peppers, diced

- 1/4 cup onion, finely chopped

- 2 eggs

- 1/4 cup low-fat cheese, shredded

- Salt and pepper to taste

Instructions:

1. In a skillet, cook ground turkey until browned.

2. Add diced bell peppers and chopped onion. Sauté until vegetables are tender.

3. Crack eggs into the skillet, sprinkle with cheese, and cover until eggs are cooked to your liking.

4. Season with salt and pepper before serving.

Nutritional Information (per serving):

- Calories: 340

- Protein: 30g

- Sodium: 320mg

- Potassium: 380mg

- Phosphorus: 280mg

19. Banana Nut Overnight Oats

Prep Time: 5 minutes (plus overnight refrigeration)

Cooking Time: 0 minutes

Serving Size: 1

Ingredients:

- 1/2 cup old-fashioned oats

- 1/2 cup almond milk (unsweetened)

- 1/2 banana, mashed

- 1 tablespoon chopped walnuts

- 1/2 teaspoon vanilla extract

Instructions:

1. In a jar, combine oats, almond milk, mashed banana, chopped walnuts, and vanilla extract.

2. Refrigerate overnight.

3. Stir before serving for a convenient and nutritious breakfast.

Nutritional Information (per serving):

- Calories: 320

- Protein: 9g

- Sodium: 60mg

- Potassium: 260mg

- Phosphorus: 120mg

20. Tomato and Basil Avocado Toast

Prep Time: 10 minutes
Cooking Time: 5 minutes
Serving Size: 1

Ingredients:

- 1 slice whole grain bread, toasted

- 1/2 avocado, mashed

- 1/2 cup cherry tomatoes, halved

- Fresh basil leaves for topping

- Drizzle of balsamic glaze

Instructions:

1. Toast whole grain bread to your liking.

2. Spread mashed avocado on the toast.

3. Top with halved cherry tomatoes and fresh basil leaves.

4. Drizzle with balsamic glaze and enjoy this vibrant and flavorful avocado toast.

Nutritional Information (per serving):

- Calories: 280

- Protein: 7g

- Sodium: 180mg

- Potassium: 400mg

- Phosphorus: 160mg

LUNCH RECIPES

1. Grilled Lemon Herb Chicken Salad

Prep Time: 15 minutes

Cooking Time: 15 minutes

Serving Size: 2

Ingredients:

- 2 boneless, skinless chicken breasts

- 1 lemon, juiced

- 2 tablespoons olive oil

- 1 teaspoon dried herbs (rosemary, thyme)

- Mixed salad greens

- Cherry tomatoes, sliced

- Cucumber, sliced

- Balsamic vinaigrette for dressing

Instructions:

1. Marinate chicken breasts in lemon juice, olive oil, and dried herbs for 10 minutes.

2. Grill chicken until fully cooked.

3. Slice grilled chicken and serve on a bed of mixed greens with cherry tomatoes and cucumber.

4. Drizzle with balsamic vinaigrette and enjoy this light and protein-packed salad.

Nutritional Information (per serving):

- Calories: 320

- Protein: 30g

- Sodium: 160mg

- Potassium: 450mg

- Phosphorus: 220mg

2. Quinoa and Vegetable Stir-Fry

Prep Time: 20 minutes
Cooking Time: 15 minutes
Serving Size: 2

Ingredients:

- 1 cup cooked quinoa

- 1 cup broccoli florets

- 1 bell pepper, sliced

- 1 carrot, julienned

- 2 tablespoons low-sodium soy sauce

- 1 tablespoon olive oil

- 1 teaspoon ginger, minced

- Sesame seeds for garnish

Instructions:

1. In a wok, heat olive oil and sauté broccoli, bell pepper, and carrot until tender-crisp.

2. Add cooked quinoa to the wok and stir-fry for an additional 2 minutes.

3. Mix in low-sodium soy sauce and minced ginger.

4. Garnish with sesame seeds and serve for a nutrient-rich and satisfying stir-fry.

Nutritional Information (per serving):

- Calories: 280

- Protein: 12g

- Sodium: 320mg

- Potassium: 350mg

- Phosphorus: 180mg

3. Lemon Garlic Shrimp Pasta

Prep Time: 15 minutes

Cooking Time: 15 minutes

Serving Size: 2

Ingredients:

- 8 ounces whole wheat pasta

- 1/2 pound shrimp, peeled and deveined

- 2 tablespoons olive oil

- 2 cloves garlic, minced

- 1 lemon, zested and juiced

- 1/4 cup fresh parsley, chopped

- Salt and pepper to taste

Instructions:

1. Cook whole wheat pasta according to package instructions.

2. In a pan, sauté shrimp in olive oil and minced garlic until pink.

3. Toss cooked pasta with shrimp, lemon zest, lemon juice, and fresh parsley.

4. Season with salt and pepper and enjoy this flavorful and kidney-friendly pasta dish.

Nutritional Information (per serving):

- Calories: 340

- Protein: 20g

- Sodium: 220mg

- Potassium: 280mg

- Phosphorus: 200mg

4. Turkey and Vegetable Skewers

Prep Time: 20 minutes

Cooking Time: 15 minutes

Serving Size: 2

Ingredients:

- 1/2 pound lean ground turkey

- 1 bell pepper, cut into chunks

- 1 zucchini, sliced

- 1 red onion, cut into wedges

- 2 tablespoons olive oil

- 1 teaspoon dried oregano

- Salt and pepper to taste

Instructions:

1. Preheat the grill or oven to medium-high heat.

2. In a bowl, mix ground turkey with dried oregano, salt, and pepper. Form into small skewers.

3. Alternate threading turkey skewers with bell pepper, zucchini, and red onion.

4. Grill or bake until turkey is cooked through and vegetables are tender.

5. Drizzle with olive oil before serving.

Nutritional Information (per serving):

- Calories: 290

- Protein: 22g

- Sodium: 120mg

- Potassium: 380mg

- Phosphorus: 220mg

5. Lentil and Vegetable Soup

Prep Time: 20 minutes
Cooking Time: 30 minutes
Serving Size: 4

Ingredients:

- 1 cup dried lentils, rinsed

- 4 cups low-sodium vegetable broth

- 1 carrot, diced

- 1 celery stalk, diced

- 1 onion, diced

- 2 cloves garlic, minced

- 1 teaspoon cumin

- 1/2 teaspoon smoked paprika

- Salt and pepper to taste

Instructions:

1. In a pot, combine lentils, vegetable broth, carrot, celery, onion, garlic, cumin, and smoked paprika.

2. Bring to a boil, then simmer for 25-30 minutes until lentils are tender.

3. Season with salt and pepper before serving.

4. Enjoy this hearty and fiber-rich lentil soup.

Nutritional Information (per serving):

- Calories: 220

- Protein: 15g

- Sodium: 320mg

- Potassium: 480mg

- Phosphorus: 220mg

6. Baked Salmon with Lemon Dill Sauce

Prep Time: 15 minutes

Cooking Time: 20 minutes

Serving Size: 2

Ingredients:

- 2 salmon fillets

- 1 lemon, sliced

- 1 tablespoon olive oil

- 1 teaspoon dried dill

- Salt and pepper to taste

- Fresh dill for garnish

Instructions:

1. Preheat the oven to 375°F (190°C).

2. Place salmon fillets on a baking sheet. Drizzle with olive oil and sprinkle with dried dill, salt, and pepper.

3. Top each fillet with lemon slices.

4. Bake for 20 minutes or until salmon flakes easily.

5. Garnish with fresh dill and serve with a side of steamed vegetables.

Nutritional Information (per serving):

- Calories: 320

- Protein: 25g

- Sodium: 120mg

- Potassium: 620mg

- Phosphorus: 280mg

7. Spinach and Feta Stuffed Chicken Breast

Prep Time: 20 minutes

Cooking Time: 25 minutes

Serving Size: 2

Ingredients:

- 2 boneless, skinless chicken breasts

- 1 cup fresh spinach, chopped

- 1/4 cup feta cheese (low-phosphorus), crumbled

- 1 clove garlic, minced

- 1 tablespoon olive oil

- Lemon wedges for serving

Instructions:

1. Preheat the oven to 400°F (200°C).

2. In a bowl, mix chopped spinach, feta cheese, minced garlic, and olive oil.

3. Cut a pocket into each chicken breast and stuff with the spinach and feta mixture.

4. Bake for 25 minutes or until chicken is cooked through.

5. Serve with lemon wedges for added flavor.

Nutritional Information (per serving):

- Calories: 280

- Protein: 30g

- Sodium: 320mg

- Potassium: 420mg

- Phosphorus: 220mg

8. Eggplant and Tomato Stew

Prep Time: 15 minutes
Cooking Time: 30 minutes
Serving Size: 4

Ingredients:

- 1 large eggplant, diced

- 1 can (14 ounces) diced tomatoes (low-sodium)

- 1 onion, diced

- 2 cloves garlic, minced

- 1 teaspoon dried oregano

- 1/2 teaspoon dried basil

- 2 tablespoons olive oil

- Salt and pepper to taste

Instructions:

1. In a pot, sauté onion and garlic in olive oil until softened.

2. Add diced eggplant, diced tomatoes, oregano, and basil.

3. Simmer for 25-30 minutes until eggplant is tender.

4. Season with salt and pepper before serving.

5. Enjoy this flavorful and low-calorie eggplant and tomato stew.

Nutritional Information (per serving):

- Calories: 180

- Protein: 3g

- Sodium: 140mg

- Potassium: 550mg

- Phosphorus: 80mg

9. Chicken and Vegetable Brown Rice Bowl

Prep Time: 15 minutes
Cooking Time: 20 minutes
Serving Size: 2

Ingredients:

- 1 cup cooked brown rice

- 1/2 pound boneless, skinless chicken breast, sliced

- 1 cup broccoli florets

- 1 carrot, julienned

- 2 tablespoons low-sodium soy sauce

- 1 tablespoon sesame oil

- Sesame seeds for garnish

Instructions:

1. In a wok, stir-fry sliced chicken until fully cooked.

2. Add broccoli and julienned carrot, stir-frying until vegetables are tender-crisp.

3. Mix in cooked brown rice, low-sodium soy sauce, and sesame oil.

4. Garnish with sesame seeds and serve for a wholesome and balanced meal.

Nutritional Information (per serving):

- Calories: 320

- Protein: 25g

- Sodium: 280mg

- Potassium: 420mg

- Phosphorus: 220mg

10. Caprese Salad with Balsamic Glaze

Prep Time: 10 minutes

Cooking Time: 0 minutes

Serving Size: 2

Ingredients:

- 2 large tomatoes, sliced

- 1 ball fresh mozzarella, sliced

- Fresh basil leaves

- Balsamic glaze for drizzling

- Olive oil for drizzling

- Salt and pepper to taste

Instructions:

1. Arrange tomato and mozzarella slices on a plate.

2. Tuck fresh basil leaves between the slices.

3. Drizzle with balsamic glaze and olive oil.

4. Season with salt and pepper and enjoy this classic and refreshing Caprese salad.

Nutritional Information (per serving):

- Calories: 280

- Protein: 15g

- Sodium: 280mg

- Potassium: 550mg

- Phosphorus: 220mg

11. Sweet Potato and Black Bean Bowl

Prep Time: 20 minutes

Cooking Time: 25 minutes

Serving Size: 2

Ingredients:

- 2 sweet potatoes, peeled and diced

- 1 can (15 ounces) black beans, rinsed and drained

- 1 teaspoon chili powder

- 1/2 teaspoon cumin

- 2 tablespoons olive oil

- Fresh cilantro for garnish

Instructions:

1. Preheat the oven to 400°F (200°C).

2. Toss diced sweet potatoes with olive oil, chili powder, and cumin.

3. Roast in the oven for 25 minutes or until sweet potatoes are tender.

4. In a bowl, combine roasted sweet potatoes with black beans.

5. Garnish with fresh cilantro and serve for a flavorful and fiber-rich bowl.

Nutritional Information (per serving):

- Calories: 320

- Protein: 10g

- Sodium: 260mg

- Potassium: 550mg

- Phosphorus: 160mg

12. Tuna and White Bean Salad

Prep Time: 15 minutes
Cooking Time: 0 minutes
Serving Size: 2

Ingredients:

- 1 can (15 ounces) white beans, drained and rinsed

- 1 can (5 ounces) tuna in water, drained

- 1/4 cup red onion, finely chopped

- 1/4 cup cherry tomatoes, halved

- 2 tablespoons olive oil

- 1 tablespoon red wine vinegar

- Fresh parsley for garnish

Instructions:

1. In a bowl, combine white beans, tuna, red onion, and cherry tomatoes.

2. Drizzle with olive oil and red wine vinegar. Toss to combine.

3. Garnish with fresh parsley and enjoy this protein-packed and satisfying salad.

Nutritional Information (per serving):

- Calories: 280

- Protein: 20g

- Sodium: 300mg

- Potassium: 480mg

- Phosphorus: 220mg

13. Roasted Vegetable Quinoa Bowl

Prep Time: 20 minutes
Cooking Time: 25 minutes
Serving Size: 2

Ingredients:

- 1 cup cooked quinoa

- 1 zucchini, sliced

- 1 bell pepper, sliced

- 1 red onion, sliced

- 2 tablespoons olive oil

- 1 teaspoon dried thyme

- Salt and pepper to taste

Instructions:

1. Preheat the oven to 425°F (220°C).

2. Toss sliced zucchini, bell pepper, and red onion with olive oil and dried thyme.

3. Roast in the oven for 25 minutes or until vegetables are golden and tender.

4. Serve roasted vegetables over cooked quinoa for a nutritious and flavorful bowl.

Nutritional Information (per serving):

- Calories: 320

- Protein: 10g

- Sodium: 20mg

- Potassium: 380mg

- Phosphorus: 180mg

14. Shrimp and Avocado Salad

Prep Time: 15 minutes

Cooking Time: 5 minutes

Serving Size: 2

Ingredients:

- 1/2 pound shrimp, peeled and deveined

- 2 avocados, diced

- 1 cup cherry tomatoes, halved

- 2 tablespoons olive oil

- 1 tablespoon lime juice

- Fresh cilantro for garnish

- Salt and pepper to taste

Instructions:

1. Sauté shrimp in olive oil until pink and cooked through.

2. In a bowl, combine diced avocados, cherry tomatoes, and lime juice.

3. Add cooked shrimp to the bowl and toss gently.

4. Garnish with fresh cilantro and season with salt and pepper.

5. Enjoy this light and refreshing shrimp and avocado salad.

Nutritional Information (per serving):

- Calories: 320

- Protein: 20g

- Sodium: 240mg

- Potassium: 620mg

- Phosphorus: 220mg

15. Chickpea and Vegetable Curry

Prep Time: 20 minutes

Cooking Time: 25 minutes

Serving Size: 4

Ingredients:

- 2 cans (15 ounces each) chickpeas, drained and rinsed

- 1 cup cauliflower florets

- 1 cup carrots, sliced

- 1 onion, diced

- 2 cloves garlic, minced

- 1 can (14 ounces) diced tomatoes (low-sodium)

- 1 can (14 ounces) coconut milk (unsweetened)

- 2 tablespoons curry powder

- 1 tablespoon olive oil

Instructions:

1. In a pot, sauté onion and garlic in olive oil until softened.

2. Add chickpeas, cauliflower, carrots, diced tomatoes, coconut milk, and curry powder.

3. Simmer for 20-25 minutes until vegetables are tender.

4. Serve this hearty chickpea and vegetable curry over brown rice.

Nutritional Information (per serving):

- Calories: 280

- Protein: 12g

- Sodium: 320mg

- Potassium: 580mg

- Phosphorus: 220mg

16. Greek Chicken Souvlaki Wrap

Prep Time: 20 minutes
Cooking Time: 10 minutes
Serving Size: 2

Ingredients:

- 1/2 pound boneless, skinless chicken breast, sliced

- 2 whole grain wraps

- 1/4 cup Greek yogurt

- 1 cucumber, sliced

- 1 tomato, sliced

- Red onion, thinly sliced

- Fresh mint leaves for garnish

Instructions:

1. Grill sliced chicken until fully cooked.

2. Warm whole grain wraps.

3. Spread Greek yogurt on each wrap and layer with grilled chicken, cucumber, tomato, red onion, and fresh mint.

4. Roll up the wraps and enjoy this Mediterranean-inspired chicken souvlaki.

Nutritional Information (per serving):

- Calories: 340

- Protein: 25g

- Sodium: 300mg

- Potassium: 420mg

- Phosphorus: 220mg

17. Mushroom and Spinach Quiche

Prep Time: 15 minutes

Cooking Time: 35 minutes

Serving Size: 4

Ingredients:

- 1 whole grain pie crust

- 1 cup mushrooms, sliced

- 2 cups fresh spinach, chopped

- 4 large eggs

- 1 cup milk (low-fat)

- 1/2 cup feta cheese (low-phosphorus), crumbled

- Salt and pepper to taste

Instructions:

1. Preheat the oven to 375°F (190°C).

2. In a skillet, sauté mushrooms and spinach until spinach is wilted.

3. In a bowl, whisk eggs and milk. Season with salt and pepper.

4. Place pie crust in a baking dish. Spread mushroom and spinach mixture over the crust.

5. Pour egg mixture over the vegetables and sprinkle with crumbled feta cheese.

6. Bake for 35 minutes or until the quiche is set.

Nutritional Information (per serving):

- Calories: 320

- Protein: 18g

- Sodium: 340mg

- Potassium: 380mg

- Phosphorus: 220mg

18. Turkey and Vegetable Lettuce Wraps

Prep Time: 20 minutes
Cooking Time: 15 minutes
Serving Size: 4

Ingredients:

- 1/2 pound lean ground turkey

- 1 cup mushrooms, finely chopped

- 1 carrot, julienned

- 1/4 cup soy sauce (low-sodium)

- 1 tablespoon sesame oil

- Lettuce leaves for wrapping

- Green onions for garnish

Instructions:

1. In a skillet, brown ground turkey until cooked through.

2. Add chopped mushrooms and julienned carrot, cooking until vegetables are tender.

3. Stir in low-sodium soy sauce and sesame oil.

4. Spoon the turkey and vegetable mixture into lettuce leaves and garnish with green onions.

Nutritional Information (per serving):

- Calories: 280

- Protein: 20g

- Sodium: 340mg

- Potassium: 420mg

- Phosphorus: 200mg

19. Ratatouille with Quinoa

Prep Time: 20 minutes
Cooking Time: 30 minutes
Serving Size: 4

Ingredients:

- 1 cup quinoa

- 1 eggplant, diced

- 1 zucchini, sliced

- 1 bell pepper, diced

- 1 onion, diced

- 2 cloves garlic, minced

- 1 can (14 ounces) diced tomatoes (low-sodium)

- 2 tablespoons olive oil

- 1 teaspoon dried thyme

- Salt and pepper to taste

Instructions:

1. Cook quinoa according to package instructions.

2. In a pot, sauté onion and garlic in olive oil until softened.

3. Add diced eggplant, sliced zucchini, diced bell pepper, diced tomatoes, dried thyme, salt, and pepper.

4. Simmer for 25-30 minutes until vegetables are tender.

5. Serve ratatouille over cooked quinoa for a delicious and wholesome meal.

Nutritional Information (per serving):

- Calories: 320

- Protein: 12g

- Sodium: 180mg

- Potassium: 620mg

- Phosphorus: 220mg

20. Blackened Tilapia Tacos

Prep Time: 15 minutes

Cooking Time: 10 minutes

Serving Size: 4

Ingredients:

- 1 pound tilapia fillets

- 2 tablespoons blackening seasoning

- 8 whole grain tortillas

- 1 cup cabbage, shredded

- 1/2 cup Greek yogurt

- 1 lime, cut into wedges

- Fresh cilantro for garnish

Instructions:

1. Coat tilapia fillets with blackening seasoning.

2. Cook tilapia in a pan over medium-high heat until blackened and cooked through.

3. Warm whole grain tortillas.

4. Assemble tacos with shredded cabbage, blackened tilapia, a dollop of Greek yogurt, and a squeeze of lime.

5. Garnish with fresh cilantro and enjoy these flavorful and healthy fish tacos.

Nutritional Information (per serving):

- Calories: 320

- Protein: 25g

- Sodium: 340mg

- Potassium: 480mg

- Phosphorus: 220mg

DINNER RECIPES

1. Lemon Herb Baked Chicken

Prep Time: 15 minutes

Cooking Time: 30 minutes

Serving Size: 2

Ingredients:

- 2 boneless, skinless chicken breasts

- 1 lemon, juiced

- 2 tablespoons olive oil

- 1 teaspoon dried herbs (rosemary, thyme)

- Salt and pepper to taste

- Fresh parsley for garnish

Instructions:

1. Preheat the oven to 375°F (190°C).

2. In a bowl, mix lemon juice, olive oil, dried herbs, salt, and pepper.

3. Place chicken breasts in a baking dish and pour the lemon herb mixture over them.

4. Bake for 30 minutes or until chicken is cooked through.

5. Garnish with fresh parsley before serving.

Nutritional Information (per serving):

- Calories: 320

- Protein: 30g

- Sodium: 160mg

- Potassium: 450mg

- Phosphorus: 220mg

2. Vegetable and Chicken Stir-Fry

Prep Time: 20 minutes

Cooking Time: 15 minutes

Serving Size: 2

Ingredients:

- 1/2 pound boneless, skinless chicken breast, sliced

- 1 cup broccoli florets

- 1 bell pepper, sliced

- 1 carrot, julienned

- 2 tablespoons low-sodium soy sauce

- 1 tablespoon olive oil

- 1 teaspoon ginger, minced

- Sesame seeds for garnish

Instructions:

1. In a wok, stir-fry sliced chicken until fully cooked.

2. Add broccoli, bell pepper, and julienned carrot, cooking until vegetables are tender-crisp.

3. Mix in low-sodium soy sauce and minced ginger.

4. Garnish with sesame seeds and serve over brown rice.

Nutritional Information (per serving):

- Calories: 340

- Protein: 25g

- Sodium: 280mg

- Potassium: 420mg

- Phosphorus: 220mg

3. Shrimp and Asparagus Quinoa Bowl

Prep Time: 15 minutes

Cooking Time: 20 minutes

Serving Size: 2

Ingredients:

- 1 cup cooked quinoa

- 1/2 pound shrimp, peeled and deveined

- 1 bunch asparagus, trimmed and cut into pieces

- 2 tablespoons olive oil

- 1 lemon, juiced

- Salt and pepper to taste

Instructions:

1. In a pan, sauté shrimp and asparagus in olive oil until shrimp are pink and asparagus is tender.

2. Toss cooked quinoa with the shrimp and asparagus.

3. Drizzle with fresh lemon juice and season with salt and pepper.

4. Serve for a light and flavorful dinner option.

Nutritional Information (per serving):

- Calories: 320

- Protein: 20g

- Sodium: 220mg

- Potassium: 380mg

- Phosphorus: 220mg

4. Mediterranean Baked Cod

Prep Time: 15 minutes

Cooking Time: 20 minutes

Serving Size: 2

Ingredients:

- 2 cod fillets

- 1 cup cherry tomatoes, halved

- 1/4 cup Kalamata olives, sliced

- 2 tablespoons olive oil

- 1 teaspoon dried oregano

- Salt and pepper to taste

- Fresh parsley for garnish

Instructions:

1. Preheat the oven to 375°F (190°C).

2. Place cod fillets in a baking dish.

3. Surround the cod with cherry tomatoes and sliced Kalamata olives.

4. Drizzle with olive oil, sprinkle with dried oregano, salt, and pepper.

5. Bake for 20 minutes or until cod flakes easily.

6. Garnish with fresh parsley before serving.

Nutritional Information (per serving):

- Calories: 290

- Protein: 25g

- Sodium: 320mg

- Potassium: 420mg

- Phosphorus: 220mg

5. Eggplant and Tomato Pasta

Prep Time: 20 minutes

Cooking Time: 25 minutes

Serving Size: 2

Ingredients:

- 8 ounces whole wheat pasta

- 1 large eggplant, diced

- 1 can (14 ounces) diced tomatoes (low-sodium)

- 2 cloves garlic, minced

- 2 tablespoons olive oil

- 1 teaspoon dried basil

- Salt and pepper to taste

Instructions:

1. Cook whole wheat pasta according to package instructions.

2. In a pan, sauté diced eggplant and minced garlic in olive oil until softened.

3. Add diced tomatoes, dried basil, salt, and pepper. Simmer for 15 minutes.

4. Toss cooked pasta with the eggplant and tomato mixture.

5. Serve for a hearty and satisfying dinner.

Nutritional Information (per serving):

- Calories: 320

- Protein: 10g

- Sodium: 220mg

- Potassium: 380mg

- Phosphorus: 180mg

6. Turkey and Vegetable Skillet

Prep Time: 15 minutes

Cooking Time: 20 minutes

Serving Size: 2

Ingredients:

- 1/2 pound lean ground turkey

- 1 zucchini, diced

- 1 bell pepper, diced

- 1 onion, diced

- 1 can (14 ounces) diced tomatoes (low-sodium)

- 1 teaspoon dried Italian herbs

- 2 tablespoons olive oil

- Salt and pepper to taste

Instructions:

1. In a skillet, brown ground turkey in olive oil until cooked through.

2. Add diced zucchini, bell pepper, and onion. Sauté until vegetables are tender.

3. Mix in diced tomatoes and dried Italian herbs. Simmer for 10 minutes.

4. Season with salt and pepper before serving.

Nutritional Information (per serving):

- Calories: 290

- Protein: 25g

- Sodium: 280mg

- Potassium: 450mg

- Phosphorus: 200mg

7. Baked Lemon Dill Salmon

Prep Time: 15 minutes

Cooking Time: 20 minutes

Serving Size: 2

Ingredients:

- 2 salmon fillets

- 1 lemon, sliced

- 1 tablespoon olive oil

- 1 teaspoon dried dill

- Salt and pepper to taste

- Fresh dill for garnish

Instructions:

1. Preheat the oven to 375°F (190°C).

2. Place salmon fillets on a baking sheet. Drizzle with olive oil and sprinkle with dried dill, salt, and pepper.

3. Top each fillet with lemon slices.

4. Bake for 20 minutes or until salmon flakes easily.

5. Garnish with fresh dill before serving.

Nutritional Information (per serving):

- Calories: 320

- Protein: 25g

- Sodium: 120mg

- Potassium: 620mg

- Phosphorus: 280mg

8. Lentil and Vegetable Stew

Prep Time: 20 minutes

Cooking Time: 30 minutes

Serving Size: 4

Ingredients:

- 1 cup dried lentils, rinsed

- 4 cups low-sodium vegetable broth

- 1 carrot, diced

- 1 celery stalk, diced

- 1 onion, diced

- 2 cloves garlic, minced

- 1 teaspoon cumin

- 1/2 teaspoon smoked paprika

- Salt and pepper to taste

Instructions:

1. In a pot, combine lentils, vegetable broth, carrot, celery, onion, garlic, cumin, and smoked paprika.

2. Bring to a boil, then simmer for 25-30 minutes until lentils are tender.

3. Season with salt and pepper before serving.

4. Enjoy this fiber-rich and protein-packed lentil and vegetable stew.

Nutritional Information (per serving):

- Calories: 220

- Protein: 15g

- Sodium: 320mg

- Potassium: 480mg

- Phosphorus: 220mg

9. Chicken and Spinach Curry

Prep Time: 20 minutes

Cooking Time: 25 minutes

Serving Size: 2

Ingredients:

- 1/2 pound boneless, skinless chicken breast, cubed

- 2 cups fresh spinach, chopped

- 1 onion, diced

- 2 cloves garlic, minced

- 1 can (14 ounces) diced tomatoes (low-sodium)

- 1/2 cup coconut milk (unsweetened)

- 2 tablespoons curry powder

- 1 tablespoon olive oil

Instructions:

1. In a pan, sauté cubed chicken in olive oil until browned.

2. Add diced onion and minced garlic, cooking until softened.

3. Stir in diced tomatoes, coconut milk, and curry powder. Simmer for 15 minutes.

4. Add chopped spinach and cook until wilted.

5. Serve this flavorful chicken and spinach curry over brown rice.

Nutritional Information (per serving):

- Calories: 280

- Protein: 20g

- Sodium: 320mg

- Potassium: 580mg

- Phosphorus: 220mg

10. Quinoa and Black Bean Stuffed Peppers

Prep Time: 20 minutes

Cooking Time: 25 minutes

Serving Size: 4

Ingredients:

- 1 cup cooked quinoa

- 1 can (15 ounces) black beans, drained and rinsed

- 1 cup corn kernels

- 1 bell pepper, halved

- 1 cup tomato sauce (low-sodium)

- 1 teaspoon cumin

- 1/2 teaspoon chili powder

- Fresh cilantro for garnish

Instructions:

1. Preheat the oven to 375°F (190°C).

2. In a bowl, mix cooked quinoa, black beans, corn, cumin, and chili powder.

3. Stuff halved bell peppers with the quinoa mixture.

4. Pour tomato sauce over the stuffed peppers.

5. Bake for 25 minutes or until peppers are tender.

6. Garnish with fresh cilantro before serving.

Nutritional Information (per serving):

- Calories: 320

- Protein: 15g

- Sodium: 180mg

- Potassium: 550mg

- Phosphorus: 220mg

11. Spinach and Feta Stuffed Turkey Meatballs

Prep Time: 20 minutes

Cooking Time: 20 minutes

Serving Size: 4

Ingredients:

- 1/2 pound lean ground turkey

- 2 cups fresh spinach, chopped

- 1/4 cup feta cheese (low-phosphorus), crumbled

- 1 egg

- 2 cloves garlic, minced

- 1/2 cup whole wheat breadcrumbs

- Salt and pepper to taste

Instructions:

1. Preheat the oven to 375°F (190°C).

2. In a bowl, combine ground turkey, chopped spinach, crumbled feta, egg, minced garlic, breadcrumbs, salt, and pepper.

3. Form the mixture into meatballs and place on a baking sheet.

4. Bake for 20 minutes or until meatballs are cooked through.

5. Serve these spinach and feta stuffed turkey meatballs with a side of steamed vegetables.

Nutritional Information (per serving):

- Calories: 280

- Protein: 25g

- Sodium: 320mg

- Potassium: 420mg

- Phosphorus: 200mg

12. Lemon Garlic Shrimp and Broccoli

Prep Time: 15 minutes

Cooking Time: 15 minutes

Serving Size: 2

Ingredients:

- 1/2 pound shrimp, peeled and deveined

- 2 cups broccoli florets

- 2 tablespoons olive oil

- 2 cloves garlic, minced

- 1 lemon, juiced

- Salt and pepper to taste

Instructions:

1. In a pan, sauté shrimp in olive oil and minced garlic until pink.

2. Add broccoli florets to the pan and stir-fry until tender.

3. Drizzle lemon juice over the shrimp and broccoli.

4. Season with salt and pepper before serving.

Nutritional Information (per serving):

- Calories: 320

- Protein: 20g

- Sodium: 220mg

- Potassium: 420mg

- Phosphorus: 220mg

13. Stuffed Acorn Squash with Quinoa and Turkey

Prep Time: 20 minutes

Cooking Time: 40 minutes

Serving Size: 4

Ingredients:

- 2 acorn squash, halved and seeds removed

- 1 cup cooked quinoa

- 1/2 pound lean ground turkey

- 1/2 cup cranberries, dried

- 1/4 cup chopped pecans

- 1 tablespoon maple syrup

- 1 teaspoon cinnamon

- Salt and pepper to taste

Instructions:

1. Preheat the oven to 400°F (200°C).

2. Place acorn squash halves on a baking sheet.

3. In a skillet, brown ground turkey. Mix in cooked quinoa, dried cranberries, chopped pecans, maple syrup, cinnamon, salt, and pepper.

4. Stuff each acorn squash half with the turkey and quinoa mixture.

5. Bake for 40 minutes or until squash is tender.

6. Enjoy these delicious stuffed acorn squash halves.

Nutritional Information (per serving):

- Calories: 340

- Protein: 20g

- Sodium: 100mg

- Potassium: 780mg

- Phosphorus: 220mg

14. Cauliflower and Chickpea Curry

Prep Time: 20 minutes
Cooking Time: 25 minutes
Serving Size: 4

Ingredients:

- 1 head cauliflower, cut into florets

- 2 cans (15 ounces each) chickpeas, drained and rinsed

- 1 onion, diced

- 2 cloves garlic, minced

- 1 can (14 ounces) diced tomatoes (low-sodium)

- 1/2 cup coconut milk (unsweetened)

- 2 tablespoons curry powder

- 1 tablespoon olive oil

Instructions:

1. In a pot, sauté diced onion and minced garlic in olive oil until softened.

2. Add cauliflower florets, chickpeas, diced tomatoes, coconut milk, and curry powder.

3. Simmer for 20-25 minutes until cauliflower is tender.

4. Serve this hearty cauliflower and chickpea curry over brown rice.

Nutritional Information (per serving):

- Calories: 280

- Protein: 12g

- Sodium: 320mg

- Potassium: 580mg

- Phosphorus: 220mg

15. Turkey and Sweet Potato Hash

Prep Time: 15 minutes

Cooking Time: 20 minutes

Serving Size: 2

Ingredients:

- 1/2 pound lean ground turkey

- 2 sweet potatoes, peeled and diced

- 1 bell pepper, diced

- 1 onion, diced

- 2 tablespoons olive oil

- 1 teaspoon smoked paprika

- Salt and pepper to taste

- Fresh parsley for garnish

Instructions:

1. In a skillet, brown ground turkey in olive oil until cooked through.

2. Add diced sweet potatoes, bell pepper, and onion. Sauté until vegetables are tender.

3. Season with smoked paprika, salt, and pepper.

4. Garnish with fresh parsley before serving.

Nutritional Information (per serving):

- Calories: 320

- Protein: 20g

- Sodium: 260mg

- Potassium: 620mg

- Phosphorus: 220mg

16. Baked Zucchini and Tomato Casserole

Prep Time: 15 minutes

Cooking Time: 30 minutes

Serving Size: 4

Ingredients:

- 3 zucchinis, sliced

- 1 cup cherry tomatoes, halved

- 1 onion, sliced

- 2 cloves garlic, minced

- 2 tablespoons olive oil

- 1 teaspoon dried basil

- Salt and pepper to taste

- 1/2 cup Parmesan cheese, grated

Instructions:

1. Preheat the oven to 375°F (190°C).

2. In a baking dish, layer sliced zucchini, cherry tomatoes, sliced onion, and minced garlic.

3. Drizzle with olive oil and sprinkle with dried basil, salt, and pepper.

4. Top with grated Parmesan cheese.

5. Bake for 30 minutes or until vegetables are tender and cheese is melted.

Nutritional Information (per serving):

- Calories: 220

- Protein: 8g

- Sodium: 260mg

- Potassium: 740mg

- Phosphorus: 160mg

17. Teriyaki Salmon with Broccoli

Prep Time: 15 minutes

Cooking Time: 20 minutes

Serving Size: 2

Ingredients:

- 2 salmon fillets

- 1 cup broccoli florets

- 2 tablespoons low-sodium teriyaki sauce

- 1 tablespoon olive oil

- 1 teaspoon sesame seeds

- Green onions for garnish

Instructions:

1. Preheat the oven to 375°F (190°C).

2. Place salmon fillets on a baking sheet. Drizzle with low-sodium teriyaki sauce and olive oil.

3. Surround the salmon with broccoli florets.

4. Bake for 20 minutes or until salmon is cooked through.

5. Garnish with sesame seeds and green onions before serving.

Nutritional Information (per serving):

- Calories: 320

- Protein: 25g

- Sodium: 320mg

- Potassium: 580mg

- Phosphorus: 280mg

18. Turkey and Vegetable Skewers

Prep Time: 20 minutes

Cooking Time: 15 minutes

Serving Size: 4

Ingredients:

- 1/2 pound lean ground turkey

- 1 zucchini, sliced

- 1 bell pepper, cut into chunks

- 1 red onion, cut into chunks

- Cherry tomatoes

- 2 tablespoons olive oil

- 1 teaspoon dried oregano

- Salt and pepper to taste

Instructions:

1. Preheat the grill or grill pan.

2. In a bowl, mix ground turkey with dried oregano, salt, and pepper. Form into small skewers.

3. Thread skewers with turkey, zucchini slices, bell pepper chunks, red onion chunks, and cherry tomatoes.

4. Grill skewers for 10-15 minutes, turning occasionally, until turkey is cooked through and vegetables are charred.

5. Drizzle with olive oil before serving.

Nutritional Information (per serving):

- Calories: 280

- Protein: 20g

- Sodium: 180mg

- Potassium: 520mg

- Phosphorus: 220mg

19. Ratatouille with Chicken

Prep Time: 20 minutes
Cooking Time: 30 minutes
Serving Size: 4

Ingredients:

- 1 pound boneless, skinless chicken thighs, cubed

- 1 eggplant, diced

- 1 zucchini, sliced

- 1 bell pepper, diced

- 1 onion, diced

- 2 cloves garlic, minced

- 1 can (14 ounces) diced tomatoes (low-sodium)

- 2 tablespoons olive oil

- 1 teaspoon dried thyme

- Salt and pepper to taste

Instructions:

1. In a skillet, brown cubed chicken in olive oil until cooked through.

2. Add diced eggplant, sliced zucchini, diced bell pepper, diced onion, minced garlic, diced tomatoes, dried thyme, salt, and pepper.

3. Simmer for 20-25 minutes until vegetables are tender.

4. Serve this delicious chicken and vegetable ratatouille over whole grain rice.

Nutritional Information (per serving):

- Calories: 320

- Protein: 25g

- Sodium: 320mg

- Potassium: 620mg

- Phosphorus: 280mg

20. Spinach and Tomato Stuffed Chicken Breast

Prep Time: 20 minutes

Cooking Time: 25 minutes

Serving Size: 2

Ingredients:

- 2 boneless, skinless chicken breasts

- 1 cup fresh spinach, chopped

- 1/2 cup cherry tomatoes, halved

- 1/4 cup feta cheese (low-phosphorus), crumbled

- 1 tablespoon olive oil

- 1 teaspoon Italian herbs

- Salt and pepper to taste

Instructions:

1. Preheat the oven to 375°F (190°C).

2. In a bowl, mix chopped fresh spinach, cherry tomatoes, crumbled feta, olive oil, Italian herbs, salt, and pepper.

3. Cut a pocket into each chicken breast and stuff with the spinach and tomato mixture.

4. Place stuffed chicken breasts on a baking sheet.

5. Bake for 25 minutes or until chicken is cooked through.

6. Enjoy these flavorful spinach and tomato stuffed chicken breasts.

Nutritional Information (per serving):

- Calories: 330

- Protein: 30g

- Sodium: 280mg

- Potassium: 480mg

- Phosphorus: 280mg

SOUP RECIPES

1. Chicken and Vegetable Soup

Prep Time: 15 minutes

Cooking Time: 30 minutes

Serving Size: 4

Ingredients:

- 1 pound boneless, skinless chicken breasts, cooked and shredded

- 1 carrot, diced

- 1 celery stalk, diced

- 1 onion, diced

- 2 cloves garlic, minced

- 6 cups low-sodium chicken broth

- 1 cup green beans, chopped

- 1 teaspoon dried thyme

- Salt and pepper to taste

Instructions:

1. In a pot, sauté diced carrot, celery, onion, and minced garlic until softened.

2. Add shredded chicken, chicken broth, chopped green beans, dried thyme, salt, and pepper.

3. Simmer for 20-25 minutes until vegetables are tender.

4. Serve this comforting chicken and vegetable soup for a kidney-friendly meal.

Nutritional Information (per serving):

- Calories: 220

- Protein: 25g

- Sodium: 280mg

- Potassium: 450mg

- Phosphorus: 200mg

2. Lentil and Spinach Soup

Prep Time: 20 minutes
Cooking Time: 35 minutes
Serving Size: 4

Ingredients:

- 1 cup dried green lentils, rinsed

- 4 cups low-sodium vegetable broth

- 1 onion, diced

- 2 carrots, diced

- 2 cloves garlic, minced

- 2 cups fresh spinach, chopped

- 1 teaspoon cumin

- 1/2 teaspoon smoked paprika

- Salt and pepper to taste

Instructions:

1. In a pot, combine lentils, vegetable broth, diced onion, diced carrots, minced garlic, cumin, smoked paprika, salt, and pepper.

2. Bring to a boil, then simmer for 30 minutes until lentils are tender.

3. Stir in chopped fresh spinach and cook until wilted.

4. Enjoy this nutrient-rich lentil and spinach soup.

Nutritional Information (per serving):

- Calories: 240

- Protein: 15g

- Sodium: 320mg

- Potassium: 580mg

- Phosphorus: 220mg

3. Tomato Basil Quinoa Soup

Prep Time: 15 minutes

Cooking Time: 25 minutes

Serving Size: 4

Ingredients:

- 1 cup quinoa, rinsed

- 1 can (28 ounces) crushed tomatoes (low-sodium)

- 1 onion, diced

- 2 cloves garlic, minced

- 4 cups low-sodium vegetable broth

- 1 cup fresh basil, chopped

- 1 teaspoon dried oregano

- Salt and pepper to taste

Instructions:

1. In a pot, sauté diced onion and minced garlic until softened.

2. Add quinoa, crushed tomatoes, vegetable broth, dried oregano, salt, and pepper.

3. Simmer for 20 minutes until quinoa is cooked.

4. Stir in chopped fresh basil before serving.

Nutritional Information (per serving):

- Calories: 280

- Protein: 10g

- Sodium: 280mg

- Potassium: 420mg

- Phosphorus: 180mg

4. Creamy Cauliflower Soup

Prep Time: 15 minutes

Cooking Time: 30 minutes

Serving Size: 4

Ingredients:

- 1 head cauliflower, chopped

- 1 onion, diced

- 2 cloves garlic, minced

- 4 cups low-sodium vegetable broth

- 1 cup unsweetened almond milk

- 2 tablespoons olive oil

- 1 teaspoon dried thyme

- Salt and pepper to taste

Instructions:

1. In a pot, sauté diced onion and minced garlic in olive oil until softened.

2. Add chopped cauliflower, vegetable broth, almond milk, dried thyme, salt, and pepper.

3. Simmer for 25 minutes until cauliflower is tender.

4. Use an immersion blender to puree the soup until creamy.

Nutritional Information (per serving):

- Calories: 200

- Protein: 8g

- Sodium: 320mg

- Potassium: 520mg

- Phosphorus: 160mg

5. Spinach and White Bean Soup

Prep Time: 20 minutes
Cooking Time: 25 minutes
Serving Size: 4

Ingredients:

- 2 cans (15 ounces each) white beans, drained and rinsed

- 4 cups low-sodium vegetable broth

- 2 cups fresh spinach, chopped

- 1 onion, diced

- 2 carrots, diced

- 2 cloves garlic, minced

- 1 teaspoon dried rosemary

- Salt and pepper to taste

Instructions:

1. In a pot, sauté diced onion, diced carrots, and minced garlic until softened.

2. Add white beans, vegetable broth, chopped fresh spinach, dried rosemary, salt, and pepper.

3. Simmer for 20 minutes until vegetables are tender.

4. Enjoy this hearty spinach and white bean soup.

Nutritional Information (per serving):

- Calories: 230

- Protein: 12g

- Sodium: 280mg

- Potassium: 480mg

- Phosphorus: 220mg

6. Chicken and Rice Soup

Prep Time: 15 minutes

Cooking Time: 35 minutes

Serving Size: 4

Ingredients:

- 1 pound boneless, skinless chicken thighs, cooked and shredded

- 1 cup brown rice, cooked

- 1 carrot, diced

- 1 celery stalk, diced

- 1 onion, diced

- 2 cloves garlic, minced

- 6 cups low-sodium chicken broth

- 1 teaspoon dried thyme

- Salt and pepper to taste

Instructions:

1. In a pot, sauté diced carrot, diced celery, diced onion, and minced garlic until softened.

2. Add shredded chicken, cooked brown rice, chicken broth, dried thyme, salt, and pepper.

3. Simmer for 25 minutes until flavors meld.

4. Serve this comforting chicken and rice soup.

Nutritional Information (per serving):

- Calories: 280

- Protein: 25g

- Sodium: 320mg

- Potassium: 520mg

- Phosphorus: 220mg

7. Minestrone Soup

Prep Time: 20 minutes

Cooking Time: 40 minutes

Serving Size: 4

Ingredients:

- 1 cup whole wheat pasta, cooked

- 1 can (15 ounces) kidney beans, drained and rinsed

- 1 can (14 ounces) diced tomatoes (low-sodium)

- 1 zucchini, diced

- 1 carrot, diced

- 1 celery stalk, diced

- 1 onion, diced

- 2 cloves garlic, minced

- 4 cups low-sodium vegetable broth

- 1 teaspoon dried oregano

- Salt and pepper to taste

Instructions:

1. In a pot, sauté diced zucchini, diced carrot, diced celery, diced onion, and minced garlic until softened.

2. Add cooked whole wheat pasta, kidney beans, diced tomatoes, vegetable broth, dried oregano, salt, and pepper.

3. Simmer for 30 minutes until vegetables are tender.

4. Enjoy this wholesome and satisfying minestrone soup.

Nutritional Information (per serving):

- Calories: 320

- Protein: 15g

- Sodium: 280mg

- Potassium: 550mg

- Phosphorus: 220mg

8. Butternut Squash and Apple Soup

Prep Time: 15 minutes

Cooking Time: 35 minutes

Serving Size: 4

Ingredients:

- 1 medium butternut squash, peeled and diced

- 2 apples, peeled and diced

- 1 onion, diced

- 2 cloves garlic, minced

- 4 cups low-sodium vegetable broth

- 1 teaspoon cinnamon

- 1/2 teaspoon nutmeg

- Salt and pepper to taste

Instructions:

1. In a pot, sauté diced onion and minced garlic until softened.

2. Add diced butternut squash, diced apples, vegetable broth, cinnamon, nutmeg, salt, and pepper.

3. Simmer for 30 minutes until squash and apples are tender.

4. Use an immersion blender to puree the soup until smooth.

Nutritional Information (per serving):

- Calories: 220

- Protein: 4g

- Sodium: 320mg

- Potassium: 480mg

- Phosphorus: 120mg

9. Broccoli and Cheddar Soup

Prep Time: 20 minutes

Cooking Time: 25 minutes

Serving Size: 4

Ingredients:

- 4 cups broccoli florets

- 1 onion, diced

- 2 cloves garlic, minced

- 4 cups low-sodium vegetable broth

- 1 cup low-fat cheddar cheese, shredded

- 1/2 cup unsweetened almond milk

- 2 tablespoons olive oil

- Salt and pepper to taste

Instructions:

1. In a pot, sauté diced onion and minced garlic in olive oil until softened.

2. Add broccoli florets, vegetable broth, almond milk, salt, and pepper.

3. Simmer for 20 minutes until broccoli is tender.

4. Stir in shredded low-fat cheddar cheese until melted.

Nutritional Information (per serving):

- Calories: 240

- Protein: 12g

- Sodium: 320mg

- Potassium: 480mg

- Phosphorus: 180mg

10. Salmon and Asparagus Chowder

Prep Time: 15 minutes
Cooking Time: 30 minutes
Serving Size: 4

Ingredients:

- 1 pound salmon fillets, cooked and flaked

- 1 bunch asparagus, trimmed and cut into pieces

- 1 onion, diced

- 2 cloves garlic, minced

- 4 cups low-sodium vegetable broth

- 1 cup potatoes, diced

- 1 cup unsweetened coconut milk

- 2 tablespoons olive oil

- Salt and pepper to taste

Instructions:

1. In a pot, sauté diced onion and minced garlic in olive oil until softened.

2. Add diced potatoes, vegetable broth, coconut milk, salt, and pepper.

3. Simmer for 25 minutes until potatoes are tender.

4. Stir in flaked cooked salmon and asparagus pieces.

Nutritional Information (per serving):

- Calories: 320

- Protein: 25g

- Sodium: 280mg

- Potassium: 620mg

- Phosphorus: 280mg

DESSERT RECIPES

1. Berry Parfait with Yogurt

Prep Time: 15 minutes

Cooking Time: 0 minutes

Serving Size: 2

Ingredients:

- 1 cup mixed berries (strawberries, blueberries, raspberries)

- 1 cup low-fat Greek yogurt

- 2 tablespoons honey

- 1/4 cup granola (low-phosphorus)

Instructions:

1. In serving glasses, layer mixed berries.

2. Spoon low-fat Greek yogurt over the berries.

3. Drizzle honey over the yogurt layer.

4. Top with a sprinkle of granola for added crunch.

5. Enjoy this refreshing and kidney-friendly berry parfait.

Nutritional Information (per serving):

- Calories: 180

- Protein: 10g

- Sodium: 70mg

- Potassium: 220mg

- Phosphorus: 120mg

2. Baked Apples with Cinnamon

Prep Time: 10 minutes

Cooking Time: 30 minutes

Serving Size: 2

Ingredients:

- 2 apples, cored and halved

- 1 tablespoon unsalted butter

- 1 teaspoon cinnamon

- 1 tablespoon honey

- 1/4 cup chopped walnuts (optional)

Instructions:

1. Preheat the oven to 375°F (190°C).

2. In a baking dish, place apple halves.

3. Dot each apple with unsalted butter.

4. Sprinkle cinnamon over the apples and drizzle with honey.

5. Bake for 30 minutes or until apples are tender.

6. Top with chopped walnuts if desired.

Nutritional Information (per serving):

- Calories: 160

- Protein: 2g

- Sodium: 0mg

- Potassium: 180mg

- Phosphorus: 30mg

3. Lemon Sorbet

Prep Time: 10 minutes

Cooking Time: 0 minutes (freezing time: 4 hours)

Serving Size: 4

Ingredients:

- 1 cup fresh lemon juice

- 1 cup water

- 1/2 cup honey

- Zest of 1 lemon

Instructions:

1. In a bowl, mix fresh lemon juice, water, honey, and lemon zest.

2. Pour the mixture into an ice cream maker and churn according to the manufacturer's instructions.

3. Transfer the sorbet to a container and freeze for at least 4 hours.

4. Scoop and serve this zesty lemon sorbet.

Nutritional Information (per serving):

- Calories: 120

- Protein: 1g

- Sodium: 5mg

- Potassium: 60mg

- Phosphorus: 10mg

4. Pineapple and Mango Popsicles

Prep Time: 10 minutes
Cooking Time: 0 minutes (freezing time: 4 hours)
Serving Size: 4

Ingredients:

- 1 cup pineapple chunks

- 1 cup mango chunks

- 1/2 cup coconut water

- 1 tablespoon agave syrup (optional)

Instructions:

1. In a blender, puree pineapple chunks, mango chunks, and coconut water until smooth.

2. Sweeten with agave syrup if desired.

3. Pour the mixture into popsicle molds and freeze for at least 4 hours.

4. Unmold and enjoy these tropical pineapple and mango popsicles.

Nutritional Information (per serving):

- Calories: 80

- Protein: 1g

- Sodium: 5mg

- Potassium: 180mg

- Phosphorus: 15mg

5. Chocolate Avocado Mousse

Prep Time: 15 minutes

Cooking Time: 0 minutes

Serving Size: 2

Ingredients:

- 1 ripe avocado

- 2 tablespoons unsweetened cocoa powder

- 1/4 cup maple syrup

- 1 teaspoon vanilla extract

- Pinch of salt

Instructions:

1. In a blender, combine ripe avocado, cocoa powder, maple syrup, vanilla extract, and a pinch of salt.

2. Blend until smooth and creamy.

3. Chill in the refrigerator for at least 1 hour.

4. Spoon into serving dishes and indulge in this rich chocolate avocado mousse.

Nutritional Information (per serving):

- Calories: 220

- Protein: 2g

- Sodium: 5mg

- Potassium: 470mg

- Phosphorus: 50mg

6. Almond Flour Banana Bread

Prep Time: 15 minutes

Cooking Time: 45 minutes

Serving Size: 8

Ingredients:

- 2 ripe bananas, mashed

- 3 eggs

- 1/4 cup unsalted butter, melted

- 1 teaspoon vanilla extract

- 2 cups almond flour

- 1/2 teaspoon baking soda

- 1/4 teaspoon salt

- 1/2 cup chopped walnuts (optional)

Instructions:

1. Preheat the oven to 350°F (180°C). Grease a loaf pan.

2. In a bowl, mix mashed bananas, eggs, melted butter, and vanilla extract.

3. Stir in almond flour, baking soda, and salt until well combined.

4. Fold in chopped walnuts if desired.

5. Pour the batter into the prepared loaf pan and bake for 45 minutes.

6. Allow to cool before slicing this almond flour banana bread.

Nutritional Information (per serving):

- Calories: 280

- Protein: 8g

- Sodium: 110mg

- Potassium: 260mg

- Phosphorus: 100mg

7. Vanilla Chia Seed Pudding

Prep Time: 5 minutes

Cooking Time: 0 minutes (chilling time: 4 hours)

Serving Size: 4

Ingredients:

- 1 cup unsweetened almond milk

- 1/4 cup chia seeds

- 2 tablespoons maple syrup

- 1 teaspoon vanilla extract

- Fresh berries for topping

Instructions:

1. In a bowl, whisk together almond milk, chia seeds, maple syrup, and vanilla extract.

2. Refrigerate the mixture for at least 4 hours or overnight, stirring occasionally.

3. Spoon the chilled chia seed pudding into serving glasses.

4. Top with fresh berries and enjoy this simple and nutritious vanilla chia seed pudding.

Nutritional Information (per serving):

- Calories: 120

- Protein: 3g

- Sodium: 60mg

- Potassium: 80mg

- Phosphorus: 80mg

8. Cinnamon Baked Pears

Prep Time: 10 minutes

Cooking Time: 30 minutes

Serving Size: 2

Ingredients:

- 2 ripe pears, halved and cored

- 1 tablespoon unsalted butter

- 1 teaspoon cinnamon

- 2 tablespoons chopped almonds (optional)

- Greek yogurt for serving

Instructions:

1. Preheat the oven to 375°F (190°C).

2. In a baking dish, place pear halves.

3. Dot each pear with unsalted butter and sprinkle with cinnamon.

4. Bake for 30 minutes or until pears are tender.

5. Top with chopped almonds if desired and serve with a dollop of Greek yogurt.

Nutritional Information (per serving):

- Calories: 180

- Protein: 2g

- Sodium: 0mg

- Potassium: 230mg

- Phosphorus: 40mg

9. Blueberry Oat Muffins

Prep Time: 15 minutes

Cooking Time: 20 minutes

Serving Size: 6

Ingredients:

- 1 cup blueberries (fresh or frozen)

- 1 cup oats

- 1/2 cup almond flour

- 1/4 cup unsweetened applesauce

- 2 tablespoons honey

- 1 teaspoon baking powder

- 1/2 teaspoon cinnamon

- 2 eggs

Instructions:

1. Preheat the oven to 350°F (180°C). Grease a muffin tin.

2. In a bowl, mix blueberries, oats, almond flour, applesauce, honey, baking powder, cinnamon, and eggs.

3. Spoon the batter into the muffin tin.

4. Bake for 20 minutes or until a toothpick comes out clean.

5. Enjoy these wholesome blueberry oat muffins.

Nutritional Information (per serving):

- Calories: 160

- Protein: 5g

- Sodium: 30mg

- Potassium: 120mg

- Phosphorus: 90mg

10. Coconut Rice Pudding

Prep Time: 10 minutes

Cooking Time: 30 minutes

Serving Size: 4

Ingredients:

- 1/2 cup arborio rice

- 2 cups coconut milk (unsweetened)

- 1/4 cup sugar

- 1/2 teaspoon vanilla extract

- 1/4 cup shredded coconut (unsweetened)

Instructions:

1. In a saucepan, combine arborio rice, coconut milk, sugar, and vanilla extract.

2. Bring to a simmer and cook for 25-30 minutes, stirring frequently, until rice is tender.

3. Stir in shredded coconut.

4. Remove from heat and let the coconut rice pudding cool before serving.

Nutritional Information (per serving):

- Calories: 240

- Protein: 2g

- Sodium: 20mg

- Potassium: 120mg

- Phosphorus: 50mg

MEAL PLANNING AND BATCH COOKING

Streamlining Your Renal Diet

Meal planning is a crucial aspect of managing a renal diet, providing a roadmap for navigating the intricacies of restricted nutrients. Streamlining this process not only eases the burden of constant decision-making but also ensures that your meals align with renal health guidelines. Let's delve into strategies for streamlining your renal diet to make it more manageable and sustainable.

When streamlining your renal diet, it's essential to begin with a solid understanding of your dietary restrictions. Consult with your healthcare professional or a registered dietitian to identify specific nutrient limitations such as sodium, potassium, and phosphorus. Armed with this information, you can then create a personalized meal plan that caters to your unique needs.

One effective approach to streamline your renal diet is to focus on simple and versatile recipes. Choose recipes that use common, easy-to-find ingredients, reducing the complexity of your grocery shopping. Opt for cooking methods like grilling, baking, or steaming, which enhance flavors without relying heavily on sodium or phosphorus-laden seasonings. This simplicity not only makes meal preparation more straightforward but also allows for greater flexibility in adjusting recipes to suit your taste preferences.

Another key aspect of streamlining your renal diet is to create a repertoire of go-to meals. Identify a selection of recipes that you enjoy and meet your dietary requirements. Having a set list of favorite meals simplifies the planning process, as you can rotate these dishes throughout the week. This not only saves time but also adds a level of predictability to your diet, making it easier to manage and adhere to.

In addition, consider utilizing meal planning apps or tools to streamline the process. These tools often allow you to input dietary restrictions and preferences, generating customized meal plans and shopping lists. This technology can be a game-changer, particularly for individuals managing complex dietary needs. By leveraging these resources, you can save time, discover new recipes, and ensure that your meals align with renal health guidelines.

Weekly Meal Planning Strategies

Effective weekly meal planning is a cornerstone of success in maintaining a renal diet. This strategy involves thoughtful consideration of your dietary restrictions, nutritional needs, and personal preferences. By dedicating time to plan your meals for the upcoming week, you gain greater control over your diet, making it easier to adhere to renal health guidelines.

Start your weekly meal planning by creating a schedule that outlines each meal and snack for the week. This schedule serves as a visual guide, helping you distribute nutrients evenly and avoid overconsumption of restricted elements. Be mindful of incorporating a variety of foods to ensure a well-balanced and nutritionally dense diet.

When planning your weekly meals, pay close attention to portion sizes. Renal diets often require strict control over nutrient intake, and portion sizes play a crucial role in achieving this control. Use measuring cups or a food scale to accurately portion out ingredients, especially those high in sodium, potassium, and phosphorus. By adhering to recommended portion sizes, you can better manage your nutrient intake and support overall kidney health.

Consider designating specific days for certain types of meals. For example, you might reserve Mondays for fish, Wednesdays for poultry, and Fridays for vegetarian options. This structure not only adds variety to your diet but also simplifies your shopping list and meal preparation. It allows you to focus on specific food groups each day, making it easier to manage your nutrient intake and stay within recommended limits.

Incorporate flexibility into your weekly meal planning. Life is unpredictable, and unexpected events may disrupt your planned meals. By having a few quick and easy recipes on hand, you can adapt to changes in your schedule without compromising your renal diet. Flexibility is key to long-term success in managing a renal diet, and it allows you to navigate social events, travel, and other situations where adhering to a strict plan may be challenging.

Take advantage of batch cooking during your weekly meal planning. Preparing larger quantities of certain recipes allows you to have ready-made meals for the week, reducing the daily cooking load. Batch cooking is particularly beneficial for staples like grains, beans, and soups, which can be portioned and frozen for later use. This not only saves time but also ensures that you always have kidney-friendly options readily available.

Batch Cooking for Convenience

Batch cooking is a powerful tool for individuals managing a renal diet. It involves preparing larger quantities of meals at once, which can then be portioned and stored for later consumption. This approach not only saves time and effort but also ensures that you consistently have access to renal-friendly meals, promoting adherence to dietary guidelines.

One of the primary advantages of batch cooking is its time-saving nature. By dedicating a specific block of time to cooking, you can prepare several meals at once, reducing the need for daily kitchen sessions. This is especially valuable for individuals with busy schedules or those who may find frequent cooking challenging. Batch cooking allows you to front-load your culinary efforts, providing convenience throughout the week.

When engaging in batch cooking, focus on recipes that freeze well and maintain their quality upon reheating. Many soups, stews, casseroles, and grains are excellent candidates for batch cooking. These dishes often improve in flavor when given time to meld, and the freezing process preserves their taste and texture. Additionally, consider investing in quality storage containers suitable for freezing to maintain the integrity of your batch-cooked meals.

Another advantage of batch cooking is the ability to control portion sizes effectively. By portioning your meals during the cooking process, you can avoid the temptation to overeat or consume excessive amounts of restricted nutrients. This precision is particularly important for individuals on renal diets, where strict adherence to recommended portion sizes is crucial for managing nutrient intake.

Batch cooking also promotes cost-effectiveness. Buying ingredients in larger quantities often allows you to take advantage of bulk discounts and reduce overall grocery expenses. Additionally, preparing meals in bulk minimizes food waste, as you can use ingredients more efficiently and avoid buying excess perishable items.

To implement batch cooking successfully, start by selecting a day or time in the week dedicated specifically to this task. Plan your meals for the upcoming week, considering recipes that align with your renal diet guidelines. Create a comprehensive shopping list to ensure you have all necessary ingredients on hand. Once you've gathered your supplies, set aside a few hours for the cooking process.

During the batch cooking session, organize your tasks efficiently. Begin with recipes that require longer cooking times, such as stews or casseroles, and use downtime, like simmering or baking, to prepare other components. Utilize multiple burners on the stove and the oven simultaneously to maximize productivity. Once the cooking is complete, allow your batch-cooked meals to cool before portioning and storing them in freezer-friendly containers.

28-DAY MEAL PLAN

Day 1:

- **Breakfast:** Overnight Oats with Berries and Almonds

- **Lunch:** Grilled Chicken Salad with Lemon-Tahini Dressing

- **Dinner:** Baked Salmon with Lemon-Dill Sauce

- **Snack:** Greek Yogurt with Berries

- **Dessert:** Berry Parfait with Yogurt

Day 2:

- **Breakfast:** Quinoa Breakfast Bowl with Almond Milk and Fresh Fruit

- **Lunch:** Lentil and Vegetable Stir-Fry

- **Dinner:** Grilled Vegetable and Chicken Skewers

- **Snack:** Hummus and Vegetable Sticks

- **Dessert:** Baked Apples with Cinnamon

Day 3:

- **Breakfast:** Chia Seed Pudding with Fresh Berries

- **Lunch:** Quinoa Stuffed Bell Peppers

- **Dinner:** Turkey and Vegetable Stir-Fry

- **Snack:** Cottage Cheese and Pineapple

- **Dessert:** Lemon Sorbet

Day 4:

- **Breakfast:** Banana and Walnut Pancakes

- **Lunch:** Turkey and Vegetable Wrap with Hummus

- **Dinner:** Quinoa and Black Bean Stuffed Bell Peppers

- **Snack:** Almonds and Dried Cranberries

- **Dessert:** Pineapple and Mango Popsicles

Day 5:

- **Breakfast:** Spinach and Mushroom Omelette

- **Lunch:** Salmon and Asparagus Quinoa Bowl

- **Dinner:** Chickpea and Spinach Curry

- **Snack:** Apple Slices with Peanut Butter

- **Dessert:** Chocolate Avocado Mousse

Day 6:

- **Breakfast:** Cottage Cheese and Pineapple Smoothie

- **Lunch:** Shrimp and Avocado Salad

- **Dinner:** Lentil Soup with Vegetables

- **Snack:** Rice Cakes with Avocado and Cherry Tomatoes

- **Dessert:** Almond Flour Banana Bread

Day 7:

- **Breakfast:** Smoked Salmon and Avocado Toast

- **Lunch:** Turkey and Sweet Potato Hash

- **Dinner:** Teriyaki Chicken with Broccoli

- **Snack:** Celery Sticks with Cream Cheese and Walnuts

- **Dessert:** Vanilla Chia Seed Pudding

Day 8:

- **Breakfast:** Blueberry Oat Muffins

- **Lunch:** Caprese Salad with Balsamic Glaze

- **Dinner:** Mediterranean Shrimp and Quinoa

- **Snack:** Trail Mix with Nuts and Seeds

- **Dessert:** Cinnamon Baked Pears

Day 9:

- **Breakfast:** Almond Flour Banana Bread

- **Lunch:** Vegetable and Brown Rice Stir-Fry

- **Dinner:** Cauliflower and Chickpea Masala

- **Snack:** Hard-Boiled Eggs with Salt and Pepper

- **Dessert:** Blueberry Oat Muffins

Day 10:

- **Breakfast:** Vanilla Chia Seed Pudding

- **Lunch:** Chicken and Vegetable Kebabs

- **Dinner:** Lemon Herb Grilled Chicken

- **Snack:** Greek Yogurt and Granola Parfait

- **Dessert:** Coconut Rice Pudding

Day 11:

- **Breakfast:** Quinoa Breakfast Bowl with Almond Milk and Fresh Fruit

- **Lunch:** Tuna Salad Lettuce Wraps

- **Dinner:** Baked Cod with Tomato and Olive Relish

- **Snack:** Greek Yogurt with Berries

- **Dessert:** Berry Parfait with Yogurt

Day 12:

- **Breakfast:** Banana and Walnut Pancakes

- **Lunch:** Quinoa and Black Bean Bowl

- **Dinner:** Sweet Potato and Black Bean Enchiladas

- **Snack:** Hummus and Vegetable Sticks

- **Dessert:** Baked Apples with Cinnamon

Day 13:

- **Breakfast:** Spinach and Mushroom Omelette
- **Lunch:** Greek Chicken Souvlaki with Tzatziki
- **Dinner:** Eggplant and Tomato Ratatouille
- **Snack:** Almonds and Dried Cranberries
- **Dessert:** Lemon Sorbet

Day 14:

- **Breakfast:** Vanilla Chia Seed Pudding
- **Lunch:** Cauliflower Fried Rice with Tofu
- **Dinner:** Lemon Garlic Shrimp with Zucchini Noodles
- **Snack:** Apple Slices with Peanut Butter
- **Dessert:** Pineapple and Mango Popsicles

Day 15:

- **Breakfast:** Chia Seed Pudding with Fresh Berries
- **Lunch:** Avocado and Black Bean Wrap
- **Dinner:** Turkey and Sweet Potato Chili
- **Snack:** Rice Cakes with Avocado and Cherry Tomatoes
- **Dessert:** Chocolate Avocado Mousse

Day 16:

- **Breakfast:** Overnight Oats with Berries and Almonds

- **Lunch:** Mediterranean Chickpea Bowl

- **Dinner:** Vegetable and Lentil Casserole

- **Snack:** Celery Sticks with Cream Cheese and Walnuts

- **Dessert:** Cinnamon Baked Pears

Day 17:

- **Breakfast:** Quinoa Breakfast Bowl with Almond Milk and Fresh Fruit

- **Lunch:** Spinach and Feta Stuffed Chicken Breast

- **Dinner:** Quinoa and Vegetable Stir-Fry

- **Snack:** Trail Mix with Nuts and Seeds

- **Dessert:** Vanilla Chia Seed Pudding

Day 18:

- **Breakfast:** Almond Flour Banana Bread

- **Lunch:** Caprese Zucchini Noodles

- **Dinner:** Grilled Tofu and Vegetable Skewers

- **Snack:** Hard-Boiled Eggs with Salt and Pepper

- **Dessert:** Coconut Rice Pudding

Day 19:

- **Breakfast:** Blueberry Oat Muffins

- **Lunch:** Chicken and Broccoli Quinoa Bowl

- **Dinner:** Baked Salmon with Lemon-Dill Sauce

- **Snack:** Greek Yogurt with Berries

- **Dessert:** Berry Parfait with Yogurt

Day 20:

- **Breakfast:** Spinach and Mushroom Omelette

- **Lunch:** Tuna Salad Lettuce Wraps

- **Dinner:** Grilled Vegetable and Chicken Skewers

- **Snack:** Hummus and Vegetable Sticks

- **Dessert:** Baked Apples with Cinnamon

Day 21:

- **Breakfast:** Banana and Walnut Pancakes

- **Lunch:** Quinoa Stuffed Bell Peppers

- **Dinner:** Chickpea and Spinach Curry

- **Snack:** Almonds and Dried Cranberries

- **Dessert:** Pineapple and Mango Popsicles

Day 22:

- **Breakfast:** Quinoa Breakfast Bowl with Almond Milk and Fresh Fruit
- **Lunch:** Shrimp and Avocado Salad
- **Dinner:** Teriyaki Chicken with Broccoli
- **Snack:** Apple Slices with Peanut Butter
- **Dessert:** Chocolate Avocado Mousse

Day 23:

- **Breakfast:** Cottage Cheese and Pineapple Smoothie
- **Lunch:** Turkey and Vegetable Wrap with Hummus
- **Dinner:** Lentil Soup with Vegetables
- **Snack:** Rice Cakes with Avocado and Cherry Tomatoes
- **Dessert:** Almond Flour Banana Bread

Day 24:

- **Breakfast:** Smoked Salmon and Avocado Toast
- **Lunch:** Turkey and Sweet Potato Hash
- **Dinner:** Quinoa and Black Bean Stuffed Bell Peppers
- **Snack:** Celery Sticks with Cream Cheese and Walnuts
- **Dessert:** Vanilla Chia Seed Pudding

Day 25:

- **Breakfast:** Blueberry Oat Muffins

- **Lunch:** Caprese Salad with Balsamic Glaze

- **Dinner:** Mediterranean Shrimp and Quinoa

- **Snack:** Trail Mix with Nuts and Seeds

- **Dessert:** Cinnamon Baked Pears

Day 26:

- **Breakfast:** Almond Flour Banana Bread

- **Lunch:** Vegetable and Brown Rice Stir-Fry

- **Dinner:** Cauliflower and Chickpea Masala

- **Snack:** Hard-Boiled Eggs with Salt and Pepper

- **Dessert:** Blueberry Oat Muffins

Day 27:

- **Breakfast:** Vanilla Chia Seed Pudding

- **Lunch:** Chicken and Vegetable Kebabs

- **Dinner:** Lemon Herb Grilled Chicken

- **Snack:** Greek Yogurt and Granola Parfait

- **Dessert:** Coconut Rice Pudding

Day 28:

- **Breakfast:** Quinoa Breakfast Bowl with Almond Milk and Fresh Fruit

- **Lunch:** Tuna Salad Lettuce Wraps

- **Dinner:** Baked Cod with Tomato and Olive Relish

- **Snack:** Greek Yogurt with Berries

- **Dessert:** Berry Parfait with Yogurt

CONCLUSION

In concluding "The Ultimate Renal Diet Cookbook for Beginners," I want to express my heartfelt hope that this culinary journey has been as enriching for you as it has been for me. Crafting this cookbook was a labor of love, born out of the desire to empower individuals navigating the complexities of renal health with delicious, accessible, and nourishing recipes.

Embarking on a renal diet doesn't have to be a daunting experience; it can be a transformative and flavorful adventure. The recipes shared throughout this book were meticulously curated to not only adhere to renal dietary guidelines but also to tantalize your taste buds and make each meal a joyous experience. From vibrant salads to hearty breakfasts, satisfying lunches, and delectable desserts, every dish was designed to harmonize with your renal health while celebrating the pleasure of eating.

Understanding the importance of renal health is the first step towards fostering a positive relationship with your body. The introductory chapters laid the foundation, shedding light on the significance of a renal-friendly diet and identifying those who stand to benefit from its principles. The comprehensive guide served as a roadmap, offering insights into renal nutrition basics, the vital nutrients to monitor, the significance of fluid balance, and decoding food labels for optimal kidney health.

Getting started with the renal diet involves a personalized approach. Assessing your dietary needs, consulting with healthcare professionals, and setting up your kitchen with renal cooking essentials were explored in depth. The guidance provided aimed to make the transition into a renal-friendly lifestyle smoother, ensuring you are well-equipped to make informed choices and relish every bite.

Delving into specific meal categories, we explored an array of tantalizing options. From salads bursting with freshness to hearty breakfasts that kickstart your day, satisfying lunches, comforting dinners, tempting snacks, and delightful desserts, the recipes were curated to meet the unique demands of a renal diet without compromising on flavor. Each recipe was a testament to the idea that a renal diet can be both health-conscious and indulgent.

Meal planning and batch cooking were presented as essential tools for simplifying your renal diet journey. By streamlining your choices and adopting weekly meal planning and batch cooking strategies, you gain not only convenience but also the freedom to savor a diverse range of kidney-friendly meals without the daily hassle.

As you explore the 28-day meal plan, my wish is for you to find joy and fulfillment in each dish. May the carefully crafted combinations of flavors, textures, and wholesome ingredients bring satisfaction to your taste buds while nurturing your renal health.

In essence, this cookbook is not just a collection of recipes; it's an invitation to embrace a lifestyle that honors your well-being without compromising on the pleasure of eating. Your journey towards optimal renal health is a personal one, and this cookbook is here to be your companion, offering guidance, inspiration, and, above all, a celebration of the profound connection between food and well-being.

Thank you for embarking on this culinary adventure with me. May your kitchen continue to be a space of creativity, nourishment, and joy as you savor the flavors of a renal diet tailored just for you. Cheers to good health and delightful meals!